Geriatric Palliative Care

Editors

MADELINE LEONG
THOMAS J. SMITH

CLINICS IN
GERIATRIC MEDICINE

www.geriatric.theclinics.com

May 2015 • Volume 31 • Number 2

ELSEVIER

1600 John F. Kennedy Boulevard • Suite 1800 • Philadelphia, Pennsylvania, 19103-2899

http://www.theclinics.com

CLINICS IN GERIATRIC MEDICINE Volume 31, Number 2
May 2015 ISSN 0749–0690, ISBN-13: 978-0-323-37597-9

Editor: Jessica McCool
Developmental Editor: Colleen Viola

Clinics in Geriatric Medicine (ISSN 0749-0690) is published quarterly by Elsevier Inc., 360 Park Avenue South, New York, NY 10010-1710. Months of issue are February, May, August, and November. Business and Editorial Offices: 1600 John F. Kennedy Blvd., Suite 1800, Philadelphia, PA 191023-2899. Periodicals postage paid at New York, NY, and additional mailing offices. Subscription prices are $280.00 per year (US individuals), $498.00 per year (US institutions), $145.00 per year (US student/resident), $370.00 per year (Canadian individuals), $632.00 per year (Canadian institutions), $195.00 per year (Canadian student/resident), $390.00 per year (international individuals), $632.00 per year (international institutions), and $195.00 per year (international student/resident). Foreign air speed delivery is included in all *Clinics* subscription prices. All prices are subject to change without notice. POSTMASTER: Send address changes to *Clinics in Geriatric Medicine,* Elsevier Health Sciences Division, Subscription Customer Service, 3251 Riverport Lane, Maryland Heights, MO 63043. Telephone: 1-800-654-2452 (U.S. and Canada); 314-447-8871 (outside U.S. and Canada). Fax: 314-447-8029. E-mail: journalscustomerservice-usa@elsevier.com (for print support) or journalsonlinesupport-usa@elsevier.com (for online support).

Reprints. For copies of 100 or more, of articles in this publication, please contact the Commercial Reprints Department, Elsevier Inc., 360 Park Avenue South, New York, New York 10010-1710. Tel.: 212-633-3874; Fax: 212-633-3820, E-mail: reprints@elsevier.com.

Clinics in Geriatric Medicine is covered in *MEDLINE/PubMed (Index Medicus), EMBASE/Excerpta Medica, Current Contents/Clinical Medicine (CC/CM),* and the *Cumulative Index to Nursing & Allied Health Literature.*

Contributors

EDITORS

MADELINE LEONG, MD
Palliative Care Fellow, Johns Hopkins Hospital, Baltimore, Maryland

THOMAS J. SMITH, MD, FACP, FASCO, FAAHPM
Director of Palliative Medicine, Johns Hopkins Medical Institutions; Professor of Oncology, Sidney Kimmel Comprehensive Cancer Center, Johns Hopkins Hospital, Baltimore, Maryland

AUTHORS

LEA BAIDER, PhD
Director, Psycho-Oncology Services, Assuta Medical Center, Tel Aviv, Israel

HARIS A. CHARALAMBOUS, BM, MRCP, FRCR
Consultant; Clinical Oncologist, The Bank of Cyprus Oncology Centre, Nicosia, The Republic of Cyprus

M. JENNIFER CHENG, MD
Staff Clinician, Pain and Palliative Care Service, Clinical Center, National Institutes of Health, Bethesda, Maryland

ELIZABETH DZENG, MD, MPH, MPhil, MS
General Internal Medicine Fellow, Division of General Internal Medicine, Program in Palliative Care, The Johns Hopkins University School of Medicine, Baltimore, Maryland; Primary Care Unit, Department of Public Health and Primary Care, University of Cambridge, Cambridge, United Kingdom

MENDWAS D. DZINGINA, MBBS, DLSHTM, MSc
Cicely Saunders Institute, King's College London, London, United Kingdom

THOMAS E. FINUCANE, MD
Professor of Medicine, Division of Gerontology and Geriatric Medicine, Johns Hopkins Bayview Medical Center, Baltimore, Maryland

AMRITA GHOSH, MD, PhD
Clinical Fellow, Pain and Palliative Care Service, Clinical Center, National Institutes of Health, Bethesda, Maryland

ANTONIO GRAHAM, DO
Fellow in Geriatrics Medicine, The Johns Hopkins University School of Medicine, Johns Hopkins Bayview Medical Center, Baltimore, Maryland

RAMZI R. HAJJAR, MD, AGSF
Associate Professor of Medicine; Director, Geriatrics Medicine and Palliative Care Service, American University of Beirut Medical Center, Beirut, Lebanon

IRENE J. HIGGINSON, BM BS, BMedSci, PhD, FFPHM, FRCP, OBE, FMedSc
Professor, Cicely Saunders Institute, King's College London, London, United Kingdom

MADELINE LEONG, MD
Palliative Care Fellow, Johns Hopkins Hospital, Baltimore, Maryland

ELIZABETH LINDENBERGER, MD
Assistant Professor, Brookdale Department of Geriatrics and Palliative Medicine, Icahn School of Medicine at Mount Sinai, New York, New York

DERRICK S. LOWERY, MD
Hospice and Palliative Medicine Fellow, Emory University School of Medicine, Atlanta, Georgia

DOMITILLA MASI, MS
Research Assistant, Engelberg Center for Health Care Reform, The Brookings Institution, Northwest, Washington, DC

OLIVIA NIRMALASARI, MD
Fellow in Geriatrics Medicine, The Johns Hopkins University School of Medicine, Johns Hopkins Bayview Medical Center, Baltimore, Maryland

KAVITA PATEL, MD, MS
Fellow and Managing Director, Engelberg Center for Health Care Reform, The Brookings Institution, Northwest, Washington, DC

RICHARD PAYNE, MD
Esther Colliflower Professor of Medicine and Divinity, The Divinity School, Duke University, Durham, North Carolina; John B. Francis Chair, Bioethics, Center for Practical Bioethics, Kansas City, Missouri

CHRISTINA M. PUCHALSKI, MD, MS, FACP, FAAHPM
Professor, Medicine and Health Sciences; Director, George Washington Institute for Spirituality and Health, The George Washington University School of Medicine and Health Sciences, Washington, DC

TAMMIE E. QUEST, MD
Department of Veterans Affairs, Decatur, Georgia; Associate Professor, Department of Emergency Medicine, Emory University School of Medicine; Director, Emory Palliative Care Center; Atlanta, Georgia

ANASTASIA ROWLAND-SEYMOUR, MD
Program in Integrative Medicine, Division of General Internal Medicine, Johns Hopkins Hospital, Baltimore, Maryland

LIDIA SCHAPIRA, MD
Associate Professor of Medicine, Department of Hematology-Oncology, Massachusetts General Hospital, Boston, Massachusetts

MICHAEL SILBERMANN, DMD, PhD
Executive Director, The Middle East Cancer Consortium, Haifa, Israel

THOMAS J. SMITH, MD, FACP, FASCO, FAAHPM
Director of Palliative Medicine, Johns Hopkins Medical Institutions; Professor of Oncology, Sidney Kimmel Comprehensive Cancer Center, Johns Hopkins Hospital, Baltimore, Maryland

LIESBETH M. VAN VLIET, PhD
Department of Palliative Care, Policy and Rehabilitation, Cicely Saunders Institute, King's College London, London, United Kingdom

JULIA C.M. VAN WEERT, PhD
Professor, Amsterdam School of Communication Research/ASCoR, University of Amsterdam, Amsterdam, The Netherlands

Contents

> This article updates the 2002 Jamie von Roenn article about "the palliation of commonly observed symptoms in older patients, including pain, neuro-psychiatric, gastrointestinal, and respiratory symptoms." When palliative care was last covered in *Clinics in Geriatric Medicine*, President George W. Bush had just signed the No Child Left Behind Act, Homeland Security was being established, Michael Jackson won the Artist of the Century Award at the American Music Awards, and gas cost $1.61 a gallon. What has changed in the last decade and a half?

> Complementary and Integrative Medicine (CIM) encompasses many diverse therapies, including natural products and mind and body practices. Use of CIM is common and can benefit patients in palliative care. However, because patients in palliative care are often frail and elderly, the clinician should consider a patient's comorbidities before recommending certain therapies, such as natural products. In this article, specific examples of CIM are provided for symptoms commonly seen in palliative care.

> Geriatrics and palliative care often overlap. This article focuses on 2 areas where the disciplines may differ in their approach. The first is planning for extreme illness and death, with explicit acknowledgment that limiting therapy might be a good idea. This situation is likely to have a different impact in the course of a routine geriatrics visit than in a palliative care context. The second is pain management, especially chronic pain. In patients with sharply limited life expectancy, the risk/benefit equation tilts easily toward narcotic use. In frail elders working to remain independent, the calculus may be quite different.

> Primary care physicians are often the first medical providers patients seek out, and are in an excellent position to provide primary palliative care. Primary palliative care encompasses basic skills including basic evaluation and management of symptoms and discussions about goals of care and advance care planning. Specialty palliative care consultation complements primary care by assisting with complex psychosocial-spiritual patient and

illnesses and reduce the overall costs of care. However, factors such as poor provider reimbursement mechanisms, inadequate formal education and training, workforce shortages, and low provider acceptance and patient engagement have created barriers to the widespread uptake of palliative care. Expanding access to these services requires their integration into new models of payment and delivery, such as Accountable Care Organizations, an overhaul of formal palliative care education and training, and improved messaging about these services to patients and providers.

The journey to excellence in palliative care practice is to recognize the three identities of patients, refine skills in assessment to understand these interrelated dimensions of personhood, and hone the practices of caring to deliver truly comprehensive and personalized care. These practices require clinicians to first connect to persons with illness on a human–human level. Being fully present and engaged with patients is critical to practicing high-quality palliative care. Clinicians must encourage and elicit the story of the illness and the life of the person experiencing the illness.

Care for elderly people with life-limiting illness cannot be delivered primarily by geriatricians or palliative care practitioners. The role of these clinicians is to help carers become adept in palliative care medicine. In a culture in which family ties run deep, the offer of palliative care from an outsider may be met with suspicion. The family bond in the Middle East is strong, but the emotional response to terminal illness may push families to request futile treatments, and physicians to comply. When palliative care is well developed and well understood, it provides a viable alternative to such extreme terminal measures.

The emergency department cares for seriously ill patients across the trajectory of illness from diagnosis to death or cure. Emergency departments participate in critical illness trajectories that include initiation of life-sustaining therapies as well as caring for patients and families in their final moments of life. Emergency clinicians are uniquely poised to identify critical palliative care interventions to be used when patients and families are most in need with respect to symptom management, decisions regarding intervention and procedures to sustain life and participate in critically important decisions regarding withdrawing and withholding nonbeneficial life-sustaining therapies.

CLINICS IN GERIATRIC MEDICINE

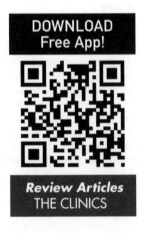

Preface

Geriatrics and Palliative Care: All in the Same Family

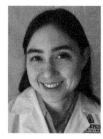 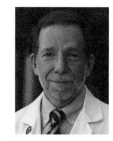

Madeline Leong, MD   Thomas J. Smith, MD, FACP, FASCO, FAAHPM
Editors

Geriatrics and palliative care (PC), officially named Hospice and Palliative Medicine, are distinct but overlapping specialties. Geriatricians do plenty of PC as they make day-to-day decisions about treating complex medical illnesses and help with advanced care planning in the elderly. However, many older patients require additional PC services, either through a PC specialist or through hospice. All the data suggest that having another team of health care professionals comanage the seriously ill patient improves quality of life, improves quality of care, may improve survival, and even lowers costs. (Our PC mantra has become "Better care at a cost we can afford.") Over 80% of hospice patients were over the age of 65 in 2012.

For these reasons, we hope that PC will be of interest to the geriatrician. In this issue, we provide education on an extensive number of PC topics: from symptom management to spirituality to public health and health care reform.

- In "Symptom Management in the Older Adult: 2015 Update," the author provides an update on how to manage common symptoms, such as pain and dyspnea.
- In "Complementary and Integrative Medicine for Older Adults in Palliative Care," the authors provide basic principles for using integrative medicine in a geriatric population, as well as recommendations for specific complementary therapies.
- In "Palliative Care in the Ambulatory Geriatric Practice," the authors discuss "planning about dying," advance directives, and chronic pain.
- In "Interaction of Palliative Care and Primary Care," the authors detail how primary care physicians can develop a "palliative care skill set" and when they should refer to specialty services.

Disclosure: Supported by P30 CA 006973, Patient Centered Outcomes Research Institute contract # 4362 (PI, Aslakson) and 1R01 CA177562-01 (PI, Ferrell).

- In "Communication with Older, Seriously Ill Patients," the authors provide a framework for empathic communication. Even though we think we have communicated, our patients often don't "get it"; for instance, only 17% of people with life-ending colorectal or lung cancer could state their prognosis correctly (<5 years and <2 years, respectively).
- In "Communications by Professionals in Palliative Care," the author offers insight into how to involve patients' families and how to conduct family meetings.
- In "Spirituality in Geriatric Palliative Care," the author explains the importance of spiritual care and provides simple, useable tools for taking a spiritual history.
- In "Public Health and Palliative Care in 2015," the authors discuss the past, present, and future of PC from a public health perspective.
- In "Palliative Care in the Era of Health Care Reform," the authors analyze the impact of the Affordable Care Act on PC.
- In "Culturally Relevant Palliative Care," the author helps us look beyond stereotypes and value cultural differences.
- In "International Palliative Care: Middle East Experience as a Model for Global Palliative Care," the authors provide case studies and field notes from the Middle East. Nearly every country in the Middle East now has a PC plan, with available opioids.
- In "Emergency Medicine and Palliative Care," the authors explain how the emergency department (ED) can be used to provide PC, since the ED is so often the entry locus for seriously ill patients, often month after month.

We are grateful to the many experts who contributed to this issue. We would also like to thank our patients, who continue to teach, inspire, and amaze us. Carpe diem.

Madeline Leong, MD
Johns Hopkins Hospital
Blalock 359
600 North Wolfe Street
Baltimore, MD 21287, USA

Thomas J. Smith, MD, FACP, FASCO, FAAHPM
Palliative Medicine
Johns Hopkins Medical Institutions
Sidney Kimmel Comprehensive Cancer Center
Johns Hopkins Hospital
Blalock 369
600 North Wolfe Street
Baltimore, MD 21287, USA

E-mail addresses:
mkunsbe1@jhmi.edu (M. Leong)
tsmit136@jhmi.edu (T.J. Smith)

Symptom Management in the Older Adult: 2015 Update

Thomas J. Smith, MD*

KEYWORDS

- Pain management • Palliative care • Pharmacologic management
- Nonpharmacologic management • Older adults • Depression • Delirium

KEY POINTS

- At least for cancer patients, being older is no longer associated with pain medication underprescribing; however, moderate to severe pain is still prevalent.
- Physician barriers include reluctance to prescribe opioids, inadequate training, fear of complications, fear of regulatory oversight, and drug interactions.
- The first principle of pain management is classification: neuropathic, and everything else.
- Symptom management continues to improve, but many more improvements are needed.

PAIN MANAGEMENT
Pain Is Still Common, and Commonly Undertreated

Dr von Roenn wrote in 2002 that, "Pain is the most common symptom for which patients seek medical attention and is one of the most frequent complaints of older adults."[1] That has not changed. The good news is that, at least for cancer patients, being older is no longer associated with pain medication underprescibing,[2] as it was in 1994. The bad news is that moderate to severe pain is still as prevalent as it was in the 1990 despite a 10-fold increase in opioid prescribing.[3]

Dr Thomas Finucane covers the important elements of pain relief elsewhere in this issue. This article reviews some of the barriers to pain and symptom management and concentrate on nonpain symptoms, in which there has been significant progress. Recent reviews of management in older adults stress the multimodality approach.[4] Barriers to pain management in older adults remain much the same as in 2002. Patient barriers include at least the following:

- Reluctance to complain
- Underreporting of pain

Disclosure: Supported by P30 CA 006973, Patient Centered Outcomes Research Institute contract # 4362 (PI, Aslakson) and 1R01 CA177562-01 (PI, Ferrell)
Palliative Medicine, Johns Hopkins Medical Institutions, Sidney Kimmel Comprehensive Cancer Center, Johns Hopkins Hospital, Blalock 369, 600 North Wolfe Street, Baltimore, MD 21287, USA
* Department of Oncology, The Johns Hopkins Hospital, 600 North Wolfe Street, Blalock 369, Baltimore, MD 21287-0005.
E-mail address: tsmit136@jhmi.edu

Clin Geriatr Med 31 (2015) 155–175
http://dx.doi.org/10.1016/j.cger.2015.01.006
0749-0690/15/$ – see front matter © 2015 Elsevier Inc. All rights reserved.

- Interpretation of pain as other words such as "discomfort"
- Reluctance to take analgesics
- Comorbidities that make prescribing more difficult
- The high cost of some pain medications, added to the cost of other medications. For instance, the price of each generic extended release oxycodone 20 mg pill is about $5, and a 75 mg pregabalin (Lyrica) capsule costs about $1.50 apiece.[5]

Physician barriers remain the same as well, including reluctance to prescribe opioids (although more patients die of complications from nonsteroidal anti-inflammatory drugs [NSAIDs] than from opioids), inadequate training, fear of complications, fear of regulatory oversight, and drug interactions.

For Pain: Classify, Classify, Classify

The first principle of pain management is classification: neuropathic, and everything else. Damage to afferent nerve fibers produces neuropathic pain, at least at the start. A distinguishing characteristic of most neuropathic pain is that it becomes amplified long after the initial insult is gone. Imagine touching a hot plate with your fingers: immediate withdrawal from the heat (mediated by the fastest, nonmyelinated Adelta fibers), then near immediate sensation of pain (mediated by the slower myelinated C fibers), then moving away from the hot plate, then blaming your son-in-law for leaving the hot plate on. Then, imagine that pain becoming worse over the next years long after the burn has healed.

Neuropathic Pain

The exact mechanisms by which neuropathic pain becomes amplified and persistent is complicated and not easily explainable. At a minimum, there are increased nerve transmitter molecules and receptor sensitivity; extra nerve "channels" or amplification along the nerve pathway, which are far more plastic than imagined 20 years ago; heightened sensitivity to chronic pain that never remits; and "wind-up" of the nerve pathways in both the spinal cord and the brain.[6] Suffice it to say that nerve pain is often out of proportion to the original pathology.

The mechanism of nerve injury matters, too. For instance, chemotherapy has become a major producer of nerve pain, chemotherapy-induced peripheral neuropathy (CIPN). Drugs like bortezomib (Velcade) used in myeloma, paclitaxel (Taxol) or eribulin (Halaven) used in breast cancer, and any platinum drug such as oxaliplatin (Oxali) used in colon cancer can cause dose-limiting neuropathy in 70% of patients. In oxaliplatin CIPN, the longest nerves actually die and drop out, leading to lowered epidermal nerve fiber density.[7] In paclitaxel neuropathy, the longest nerves are damaged, with up to 25% of the damage happening in the year after the chemotherapy has stopped, but the nerves may recover. In diabetic nerve damage, the nerve death and damage seems to be nutritional rather than toxic, but the nerves are still dead or damaged.

Neuropathic pain is also easy to "score" with the 0 to 10 scale, just like usual pain. Remember to ask all the important questions for billing (and for patient care!): when did it start, what brings it on, what relieves it, what does it feel like, and are there any associated symptoms? Neuropathic pain is typically described as sharp, burning, itching, or hot, with associated numbness and tingling. If life were fair, nerves that were absent or damaged would just give numbness, but all too often numbness and tingling are associated with the worst nerve pain. There are useable, validated research scales such as the European Organization for Research and Treatment of Cancer CIPN-20 or the DN4 questionnaire, but they are not in widespread use outside of clinical trials.[8]

We think it is more important to classify the pain as neuropathic and ask, "How is the pain limiting your activities?"

The physical examination is critical for neuropathic pain. First, allodynia (a painful impulse felt after normal touch, like brushing the skin), and second, because of the success of local nerve blocks with local anesthetics such as lidocaine or bupivicaine. If the pain can be localized to a single or localized pain generator or ganglion, then it has a good chance of being blocked. Examples include occipital nerve neuropathy or pancreas cancer pain that can be treated with a local celiac or splanchnic plexus block in 75% of cases.

Neuropathic pain is treated differently from usual somatic pain: we try to quiet down the damaged nerves with antiseizure drugs or other neuroleptics, slowly, over weeks and months. Commonly used agents include tricyclic antidepressants (desipramine, nortriptyline), anticonvulsants (pregabalin, gabapentin, carbamazepine, valproic acid), and topical agents (lidocaine, capsacian). This is a critical teach-back moment for practitioners, because the patient must know this is a long-term strategy to allow the damaged nerve to stop "pinging" and to allow normal nerves to regrow. Neuroleptic drugs are not good pain killers by themselves, so the patient must be encouraged to give the drug at least a 1-month trial, even if they do not feel any relief.

The actual treatment of neuropathic pain should be relatively simple (**Table 1**). The largest randomized trial showed that the combination of an opioid (morphine) and a neuroleptic (gabapentin) was more effective than either alone.[9] We make the assumption that this holds true for any opioid and any neuroleptic, but evidence is scant. In fact, a Cochrane Systematic Review concluded that there was no evidence that oxycodone had any sustained effect on neuropathic or fibromyalgia pain, and the usual harms[10]; however, other expert review panels concluded there was enough evidence of benefit.[11]

We also often hear that methadone is the best opioid for neuropathic pain; however, but the evidence is lacking. The one large randomized trial in cancer patients showed that morphine and methadone were equivalent in the relief of neuropathic pain, but the number of patients was too small to rule out some additional benefit.[12]

Our advice is to pick a neuroleptic drug that is safe and affordable for your patient (starting with gabapentin or pregabalin as the usual first choice[13]), escalate to pain relief or the maximum tolerated dose, and convince the patient to try it for at least 4 to 6 weeks.[14] If not successful, start again with a different drug. Many of us do not have the experience, patience, or time to do these sequential drug trials, so referral to a chronic pain specialist may be helpful. Using a simple algorithm with proven drugs, neuropathic pain could be promptly and significantly reduced in nearly all cancer patients, from 5.4 out of 10 to 2.8 out of 10 at 12 weeks.[15]

Somatic pain is well-described in Dr Finucane's article. As Dr von Roenn described in 2002:

> The initial approach to a patient with pain begins with a comprehensive pain assessment, including a thorough history of the pain, its impact on activities, and prior therapeutic interventions and their outcomes; a complete physical examination; review of all medications; and evaluation of functional status. Older patients may present with atypical manifestations of pain, including delirium, confusion, fatigue, social withdrawal, and depression. Additionally, screening for depression and anxiety is important because either state can augment the pain response and interfere with pain control.

The general approach to pain and associated symptoms is the same today an in 2002. We use a single question for depression screening, "Are you depressed?" or

Table 1
Treatment of neuropathic pain

Condition	Drug Choices	Evidence	Comments
Diabetic neuropathy	Gabapentin or pregabalin	Randomized clinical trials	Gabapentin is much less expensive (pennies vs dollars), can cause sedation and edema, and has a ceiling effect at 2700 mg/d. Pregabalin has no upper limits of absorption, but may have more psychiatric effects.
Shingles "postherpetic pain"	Prevention (early treatment) with gabapentin[16] or pregabalin[17]	Randomized clinical trials, but not in geriatric patients	The data are compelling for a single gabapentin dose of 900 mg, or pregabalin 150 mg at the outset of a shingles outbreak. The author suggests a lower dose in older adults.
Shingles "postherpetic pain"	Treatment with topical lidocaine, capsaicin, or oral gabapentin or pregabalin	Randomized, clinical trials	Excellent recent review emphasized that the elderly had the most prevalence and side effects of treatment, one-half of patients still have pain, and opioids are not usually effective.[18]
CIPN	Prevention of oxaliplatin neuropathy: venlafaxine	Randomized, clinical trial	One study with 62 patients[19] showed a significant delay and/or reduction in CIPN.
CIPN	Treatment Only duloxetine has proven efficacy; venlafaxine, a similar generic drug, is likely to work as well	One successful randomized, controlled trial Multiple failed drugs	Duloxetine reduced pain scores from 6/10 to 5/10 at 6 wk, with acceptable toxicity.[20] Generic venlafaxine may have similar activity, and the clinical trial data are forthcoming. Most of the drugs used for diabetic neuropathy do not work for CIPN, including gabapentin, nortriptylline, and lamotrigine.[21]
All others	Use an opioid if the pain is severe		The combination is better than either class of drug alone.

Abbreviation: CIPN, chemotherapy-induced peripheral neuropathy.
Data from Refs.[16–21]

"Are you bothered by depression?" to remind ourselves to assess this on every visit. Although not perfect, single-question screening has good reliability in most populations and is better than no screening tool at all.[22,23] Delirium is also more prevalent in older patients and requires a separate screening tool.

We have sequentially modified our "rounding tool" from that used in a large, multi-institutional study to the current very short form (**Table 2**). The advantage is that this reminds us to ask the questions, and each question has some readily available fixes. We import this as a Smart Phrase into EPIC, and the boxes let us add the most important questions. For instance, if the patient is depressed, we will directly ask, "What makes you most depressed?" and explore the topic fully. Our group has subsequently attempted to standardize responses to such patient reported outcomes; for each symptom, the practice should have a standard approach.[24]

Nonpharmacologic Techniques

Nonpharmacologic techniques can be an integral component of pain management. Even if they do not work fully, they may allow a lower opioid dose or allow the patient to have more control over the situation. We give some examples in **Table 3**.

PHARMACOLOGIC PAIN MANAGEMENT
Special Considerations in Older Adults

Dr Finucane outlines many of the relevant parts of the aging process and pain medications in his article. Some additional considerations, based on our experience, include the following:

- Renal function declines with each year and decade, and the risk of NSAID-induced renal failure is greater. For many older adults, muscle mass is diminished so that the creatinine is artificially low.
- Liver function declines less than renal function unless there are other liver illnesses and is easier to estimate based on the liver function tests.
- Cachexia and lower fat stores means that fentanyl transdermal will not be absorbed as well. It still works, and is the least constipating of all the opioids, but a cachectic person may need almost double the expected dose.[32]
- For moderate or severe pain, opioids are the drugs of choice. Start low and escalate the dose over days, not hours.
- Blood levels of opioids bear almost no correlation with pain relief.
- For the person in acute pain, intravenous in-hospital titration with conversion to oral doses once stable is faster than outpatient oral management.
- The prescribing hand that forgets to write the bowel regimen when prescribing the opioid is the hand that gets to do the disimpaction.

Nonopioids

Tramadol is available worldwide, inexpensive, and equal to low-dose morphine.[33] It has characteristics of both antidepressants and opioids, and should be used in caution with selective serotonin reuptake inhibitor and selective norepinephrine reuptake inhibitor drugs at the risk of causing serotonin syndrome. However, it is generally well-tolerated, has some proven efficacy in neuropathic pain,[34] and can be useful where opioids are not wanted. The starting dose is 50 mg twice a day with a maximum of 300 mg. We teach pain relief around the world in ELNEC and had to add a module for tramadol because it is uniformly available, inexpensive, and has none of the stigma of opioids. Tapentadol (Nucynta) has a similar mechanism

Table 2
An abbreviated symptom scale

| | | Reported by: Patient/Caregiver/RN/MD | | | | | | | |
| | | Able to Respond: Yes/No | | | | Delirious: Yes/No (No Benzodiazepines! Use Haloperidol) | | | |
	Pain	Tiredness	Nausea	Depression	Anxiety	Drowsiness	Anorexia	Constipation	Dyspnea	Secretions
0			X	X						X
1						X				
2										
3										
4		X exertional only		X "leaving my grandkids"	X "dying"		X	X	X exertion	
7										

Enter: 0 = none, 1 = a little bit, 2 = somewhat, 3 = quite a lot, 4 = very much, 7 = refused.
NB. Always ask "Are you bothered by _____?"

Table 3
Nonpharmacologic techniques

Method	Indication	State of the Evidence	Comment
Cognitive–behavioral interventions	Pain	RCTs, not in geriatrics	Hard to find providers Hard to convince patients to go May not be reimbursed
Acupuncture	Pain Nausea Arthralgia associated with chemotherapy or hormonal agents	RCTs RCTs RCTs	Hard to evaluate providers May not be reimbursed
TENS	Muscle pain—modestly effective Cancer pain or bone pain—ineffective	RCTs, small and underpowered	Not enough evidence to recommend[25]
Cold/heat			
Topical menthol for neuropathic pain[26]			
Promising but unproven treatments			
Scrambler therapy for neuropathic pain	Chemotherapy induced cancer pain[27,28] Postherpetic pain[29] Neuropathic pain[30]	No RCTs yet reported >50% pain relief within days, lasting months	FDA cleared, but not reimbursed by most insurers No toxicity
High-intensity light therapy	Diabetic neuropathy	RCT showed some relief of pain and dramatic return of normal function[31]	No toxicity Not readily available

Abbreviations: FDA, US Food and Drug Administration; RCT, randomized, controlled trial; TENS, transcutaneous electrical stimulation.
Data from Refs. [26–30].

of action (agonist of the μ-opioid receptor and norepinephrine reuptake inhibitor) and efficacy[35] but is expensive at $3 to $9 per pill.

Acetaminophen remains the drug of choice for mild pain, as it was in 2002. It works on the cyclooxygenase-2 receptors in the brain, and has a different mechanism of action than all the other agents, so is useful in pain management. I tell people we are building a layer cake of pain relief: we can use layers of acetaminophen, NSAIDs if safe, opioids, and nerve drugs until we get the pain down to 4 or less. Above 6, most patients will be thinking of little else than their pain; at 4 or below, the pain is tolerable. Patients should stay well below the 4 g/d prohibition, and may need to count all their "Nyquil" and other drugs.

NSAIDs have changed markedly since 2002, when there was great excitement about celecoxib (Celebrex), rofecoxib (Vioxx), and valdecoxib (Bextra) as safer cyclooxygenase-2 inhibitors. Currently, only celecoxib is in common use and can be helpful for patients in whom other NSAIDS are ineffective or contraindicated.

Corticosteroids reduce edema, and are used as adjuvant analgesics despite lack of a robust evidence base. In our own practice, we use them for liver pain, liver capsule pain, and bone pain (avoiding concurrent NSAID use). The right dose is not known for any of these indications, so we give 4 to 16 mg in 1 daily dose in the morning to avoid late-day sleeplessness.

Opioids

As in 2002, "Opioids remain the cornerstone of pain management and are the preferred agents for moderate-to-severe pain. A weak opioid is appropriate for acetaminophen-unresponsive mild pain in a patient not considered a candidate for NSAIDs. Opioids alleviate pain for most patients." Nothing has changed since then. We can make several generalizations:

- Geriatric patients may be reluctant to take opioids, until they find relief from them. Make sure you tell people that "fuzziness," nausea, and itching are common with the first several days but wear off.
- Start with half the dose you would give a 40-year-old patient, for example, oxycodone 2.5 mg every 4 hours rather than 5 mg. It is easier to titrate up than to convince a patient to retry the drug that made him sleep for 3 hours.
- All the common short-acting drugs work for 3 to 4 hours, so it makes no sense to write a prescription saying every 6 hours.
- Remember to start a bowel regimen.
- If patients are needing several daily doses, consider a long-acting drug. There are no comparative studies of long-acting morphine plus short-acting oxycodone versus the opposite, so stick with one drug for the immediate-acting and long-acting drugs.
- That said, everyone's opioid receptors are different, and we have many patients who do well with long-acting fentanyl and immediate release oxycodone. Just do not have them on 3 different long acting drugs; maximize 1 drug.
- Do not use meperidine (Demerol), propoxyphene (Darvon), or pentazocine (Talwin), a mixed agonist/antagonist.
- If patients are on a long-acting drug, make sure they have an immediate release ("rescue") drug available at about 10% of the daily dose of the long-acting drug. For example, someone on 300 mg of daily oral long-acting morphine should be on 30 mg as the short-acting dose, not 10 mg.
- Use an opioid calculator to recommend dose adjustments. Examples are http://www.globalrph.com/narcoticonv.htm and http://clincalc.com/opioids/.

Methadone

- Use methadone if you have experience using it. It is a wonderful long-acting opioid, but patients show wide variability to its effects, and respiratory depression is possible.
- Start low and titrate doses no more than every 3 days unless you have experience and a highly opioid-tolerant patient.
- Check an electrocardiogram to make sure the QTc interval is normal before starting. Many of the new cancer and cardiac drugs also effect the QTc interval. Although torsade de pointes and ventricular fibrillation are rare, they could be preventable.[36]

SPECIFIC PAIN SITUATIONS COMMON IN OLDER ADULTS
Myofascial Pain

Myofascial pain is pain owing to overuse, or just use, when joints and muscles are not as young as they used to be. Since 2002, there have been substantial strides in both treatment and evidence. The data are clear that topical NSAIDs are beneficial.[37] Derry and colleagues[37] focused on studies lasting longer than 8 weeks and found that "Topical NSAIDs were significantly more effective than placebo for reducing pain owing to chronic musculoskeletal conditions." There was an increase in local adverse events (mostly mild skin reactions) with topical NSAIDs compared with placebo or oral NSAIDs, but no increase in serious adverse events. Gastrointestinal adverse events with topical NSAID did not differ from placebo, but were less frequent than with oral NSAIDs. Mild skin reactions were more common than with oral drugs, but there was less gastrointestinal and renal toxicity. These findings fit with previous research that shows the concentration of NSAIDS in the joint fluid is substantially higher than in the blood.

Topical Patches

Lidocaine 5% topical patches (Lidoderm) also helped myofascial pain syndrome of the upper trapezius in a randomized, double-blind, placebo-controlled study—somewhat.[38] (These may be very useful for people who have contraindications to NSAIDs. The primary endpoint, pain in the shoulder and neck, improved over 14 days compared with placebo, with less neck disability. However, at 28 days there was no difference between placebo and lidocaine patches.)

Metastatic Bone Pain: Prevention

The outlook of cancer patients has changed slowly but surely since 2002, when it comes to bone metastases. When I was in intern in 1979, the wards were full of patients with fractured femurs or hips and a calcium of 16. Now, both are half as common. The big advance has been bone-modifying agents,[39] first the bisphosphonates (pamidronate then zoledronic acid [Zometa], followed by RANK-ligand inhibitors [denosumab, Xgeva]).[40] Given to patients with solid tumors and bone metastases, the risk of a "skeletal related event" (fracture, need for surgery, or radiation therapy) has been cut by more than one-half.[41] These drugs were initially given every month until the patient died, but recent randomized trials show that once-monthly treatment for a year, followed by every-3-month treatment is as effective. Denosumab is slightly more effective than the bisphosphonates, but the cost may be prohibitive for some patients and insurers. Denosumab is a single monthly subcutaneous injection, versus a 20-minute intravenous infusion.

The precautions with the drugs are the same. Renal failure with a creatinine over 3 is a relative contraindication, but if caused by hypercalcemia may be necessary. Osteonecrosis of the jaw has been increasingly recognized since the mid 2000s, and happens to 1 or 2 of 100 people who receive these drugs. It presents as an open, nonhealing ulcer down to the mandible or maxilla, often where was trauma such as radiation or a recent extraction. The exact mechanism has not been determined fully, but risk is proportional to the length of time on these drugs and the total doses.

Metastatic Bone Pain: Treatment

Successful management of metastatic bone pain demands a multidisciplinary approach, just like it did in 2002, with the same list of "systemic analgesics, bisphosphonates, radiopharmaceuticals, and external beam radiation therapy." It is critical that patients with bones at risk for a pathologic fracture (a long bone with $\geq$20% loss of the cortical bone, or >3 cm long, or a vertebrae) be evaluated by an orthopedic surgeon.

Pain relief is still critical to treatment, starting with NSAIDs and steroids, followed by opioids. Recognize that the pain while moving will be worse than the pain while being still, and give patients a breakthrough medication to take 15 minutes before they have to get out of bed or go to physical therapy (see "Incident Pain").

Radiation therapy for bone metastases has changed dramatically in the rest of the world but not so much in the United States. All the relevant guidelines call for, if feasible, a single large dose (8 Gy) of radiation ("hypofractionation") instead of the traditional 10 or more smaller fractions. This is based on numerous randomized, clinical trials showing equivalent bone pain relief, and the need for 1 consultation and treatment rather than visits for consultation, simulation, and 10 treatments. In addition, the cost to society is one-half as much. However, the revenue to radiation oncologists is similarly cut substantially. Some radiation oncologists will argue that 1 in 8 survivors will need retreatment (meaning 7 of 8 do not), but there is now compelling data that show a single, large fraction of retreatment works just as well as longer regimens. Schuster JM and colleagues[42] have taken this 1 step further: for hospice patients, they simulate and treat in 1 session for $400 total, and had 100% relief of pain in a small series.

The use of radiopharmaceuticals has increased since 2002, but only for cancer patients. These only work for osteoblastic metastases, not osteolytic holes such as with myeloma, because the radioactive technetium is taken up by macrophages involved in inflammation. The radioactive molecule replaces calcium in the bones, and gives a radioactive particle path of less than 1 cm, so surrounding tissue is uninvolved. The marrow is radiated so anemia and thrombocytopenia are the most common side effects. The most common use is for patients with multiple bone osteoblastic metastases where pain relief can be obtained within 48 hours and last for 3 to 6 months. The most recent addition, Ra 233, actually improves the average survival by 3 months from 11 to 14 in patients with metastatic prostate cancer.

Incident Pain

Mercadante has shown that "incident pain," or pain with movement from bone metastases, is exceedingly difficult to control with any measure other than radiation. The most common dose of morphine for incident pain, rapidly titrated intravenously on day 1, was 102 mg when converted to oral doses.[43] More recently, the same group has shown excellent response of incident pain to coadministered ketamine and switching the opioid to methadone, but the study was only 2 patients.[44] Incident pain was also relieved in 1 patient with a bisphosphonate infusion as part of the initial therapy,[45] but this study has not been replicated.

MISCELLANEOUS BOTHERSOME SYMPTOMS
Itching

One word: gabapentin. Gabapentin works for itching owing to burns, histamine release from hematologic malignancies, cancer, uremia, and most other pruritis.[46,47] However, gabapentin does not help pruritis owing to liver disease and bile cholestasis. Paroxetine (Paxil) at 10 mg/d was rapidly successful in 3 Japanese patients[48] and in my own practice. Sertraline (Zoloft) was highly successful in small randomized trials compared with placebo for cholestatic pruritis, and is safe and now generic.[49]

Cough

The breakthrough clinical trial was the use of gabapentin for chronic idiopathic cough. Compared with placebo, gabapentin reduced cough intensity and frequency and the cough-quality-of-life score by one-half.[50] Gabapentin has not been tested for the cough associated with pleural effusion, bronchiectasis, or idiopathic pulmonary fibrosis, but the central mechanism of action should still hold in at least some of these cases.[51] The usual doses, 300 mg/d to start (100 mg in frail patients) escalating to 1800 mg, are used.

Hiccups

There are no new clinical trials and no good evidence behind any of the interventions we try. We trial baclofen, prochlorperazine or other zines, and benzodiazepines.

Fatigue

There are 2 interventions with high-power, randomized, clinical trials to back their use: American ginseng and dexamethasone in those near the end of life. There are several trials of psychostimulants in cancer-related fatigue that show mixed and mostly negative results.

Barton and colleagues[52] at the Mayo Clinic did a pilot trial, then a large randomized trial of American ginseng at 0 mg (placebo), 2000 mg, and 4000 mg/d in patients with chemotherapy-related fatigue. The side effects were the same in all 3 groups. There was no effect on mental fatigue, but physical fatigue improved enough to be clinically important at 4 and 8 weeks. The mechanism of action of ginseng is unknown, but it may be antiinflammatory and restorative. They used American ginseng from Wisconsin, purchased at the Ginseng and Herb Cooperative (http://www.ginsengherbco-op.com/) at about $14 for a month supply. The evidence for other types of ginseng such as Siberian or Korean is less robust, and less robust for other conditions than cancer-related fatigue.

Bruera and colleagues at M. D. Anderson Cancer Center studied dexamethasone 4 mg twice a day versus placebo for 2 weeks in patients with advanced cancer. Fatigue was reduced clinically and significantly, global quality of life was improved, appetite was improved, and side effects were the same with placebo.[53] This has become our "go to" drug for rapid improvement in quality of life and energy in the last 3 months of life, as long as diabetes is not a problem.

The use of psychostimulants such as methylphenidate in cancer patients has been disappointing. Promising uncontrolled trials[54] led to larger, negative, randomized, placebo-controlled trials with methylphenidate in breast cancer patients[55] or in general cancer patients, except those with very high level of fatigue.[56] Similarly, modafinil, which is effective in multiple sclerosis had no effect in advanced cancer patients,[57] leading authorities to recognize that psychostimulants cannot overcome somatic fatigue.[58] The 1 promising aspect of these studies has been that the response to the first day of methylphenidate is highly predictive of eventual effect,[59] so a patient can be "trialed" with a 5-day supply and only continue if it works for her or him.

RESPIRATORY SYMPTOMS
Dyspnea

Dyspnea, the uncomfortable awareness of breathing, is common in palliative care and up to 75% of patients experience it near the end of life. Dyspnea is common no matter the underlying terminal diagnosis.[60] We routinely differentiate dyspnea—trouble breathing—from hypoxia and low oxygen saturation. Some patients have extreme dyspnea with 98% oxygen saturation, and others will be comfortable with 82%. Because oxygen represents another tether upon which to trip, and can cost $25 to $250 a day in the hospital or with home hospice, it should only be provided when needed.

The evidence base on which to choose therapy has expanded in the last decade. A 2008 meta-analysis of 134 cancer patients with dyspnea failed to show any benefit to oxygen therapy.[61] Abernethy and colleagues[62] subsequently randomized 239 patients with dyspnea and Pao_2 of greater than 55 mm Hg to 7 days of oxygen or room air, and found no meaningful difference in any measure; of note, dyspnea decreased with both oxygen and room air.

There is some variation in the usefulness of oxygen according to the underlying disease. In patients with chronic obstructive pulmonary disease and symptomatic dyspnea, but without hypoxemia, medical oxygen therapy does have beneficial effect, even in those who would not traditionally qualify for oxygen treatment.[63] The effect is in breathlessness and fatigue, with no discernible benefit on survival.[64]

Opioids remain as the mainstay of dyspnea treatment, as they have been for 2000 years,[65] even though the clinical trial evidence for most situations is lacking.[66] The basic science understanding has increased with the discovery of endogenous opioids (endorphins). In an elegant experiment, investigators showed the important of endogenous opioids by giving naloxone (Narcan) to dyspneic patients, and worsened their dyspnea.[67] We start patients on extremely low doses of oxycodone or morphine, 2.5 to 5 mg every 4 hours. If patients have benefit, we will try 10 mg of extended release morphine as done by Currow and colleagues[68] in Australia. At least one-third of patients achieved clinical benefit that was long lasting, although constipation was a problem even with prophylactic senna.

There may be a role for benzodiazepines in the treatment of dyspnea, but the evidence is slim. In a recent study, investigators added clonazepam 0.5 mg at night to extended release morphine in the morning for 15 chronic obstructive pulmonary disease patients. The treatment was safe and seemed to have some benefit, so larger randomized trials are ongoing.[69]

We and others have investigated inhaled nebulized medications for dyspnea, because they are preferred by most patients,[70] but the randomized clinical trial evidence is still lacking.[71] Morphine seems not to work any better than placebo. Inhaled nebulized fentanyl seemed to benefit patients in an uncontrolled study,[72,73] so a randomized trial is ongoing.

Pulmonary Secretions

Hospice and palliative medicine professionals try to prevent or treat the "Death Rattle" or secretions in the back of the throat because it is so distressing to all involved. We typically start with a scopolamine transdermal patch every 3 days, then give scopolamine or glycopyrolate in the same doses we would give in the operating room. We, as did professionals and caregivers in the UK, often feel pressured to "do something!" even if we know it is unlikely to help.[74] However, the evidence behind any of these interventions is lacking. Mercadante reviewed 11 randomized trials and found no clear-cut evidence of effectiveness of these measures as treatment modalities.[75] An even more comprehensive systematic review of 99 studies found a high prevalence, but no evidence of benefit for any intervention.[76] In addition, scopolamine 0.43 mg subcutaneously caused significant psychomotor slowing, but no effect on cognition or memory, in elderly patients compared with 10 younger patients so it should be used with caution[77]—if psychomotor slowing is an issue. A more realistic approach is to reassure the family that the patient is not suffering, position the patient for maximum comfort, and offer therapeutic presence with or without drugs.[78]

NEUROPSYCHIATRIC SYMPTOMS
Depression

Depression remains underdiagnosed and undertreated. As discussed, we use a single question screening method, "Are you depressed?" or "Are you bothered by depression?" as a way to start the assessment. It is essential to differentiate some situations that masquerade as depression:

- Fatigue (physical causes)
- Sleep deprivation
- Apathy
- Sadness (for many reasons including serious illness, isolation, etc)
- Loneliness
- Demoralization (loss of morale, or the will to continue, owing to medical or other issues).

The fixing of each of these issues requires more than a pill and rearrangement of brain biochemistry, although treatment of depression may help each situation. Treatment of depression in older adults is the same as in younger adults, with no significant changes in the last decade. We have listed some of the common treatments in **Table 4**.

Delirium

There are several decisions to make about delirium: diagnosis, evaluation, and treatment. The diagnosis should be straightforward: delirium is an acute disturbance in consciousness, cognition, and attention. It is among the most common symptoms, and can be the most upsetting to families. We use the Confusion Assessment Method (CAM) routinely[82] (having learned from our nurse colleagues in intensive care), especially Feature 4, although there are other measures (**Box 1**).

Evaluation depends on the goals of the patient and family, the expected lifespan estimated with the palliative performance scale (very accurate when the person is bedbound[83]), and our estimation that a correctable cause can be identified. We first look at all the medications, and especially at opioids (especially sudden discontinuation leading to withdrawal), steroids, antidepressants, sleep aids such as quietipine or mirtazapine, and any benzodiazepine. It is important to let the family know that the effects of the medicines may take several days to wear off. If we treat delirium, we start with a standardized approach:

- Family or a sitter at the bedside.
- Orientation and reorientation.

Table 4
Treatment of depression

Therapy	Usefulness	Additional Considerations
Cognitive–behavioral treatment	High	May be difficult to find, or be reimbursed, or convince patients to go, but well worth it.
Psychotherapy	High	
Drug treatment: antidepressants	High—the same as with other groups of patients The side effects are the same, too: energizing, sleeplessness, too much sleep, lack of sex drive/libido, and weight gain.	Try to treat other symptoms at the same time. Trazadone (Desyrel) is useful for insomnia. Mirtazapine (Remeron) is commonly used for nausea, insomnia, and appetite stimulation, despite a lack of randomized trials.
Psychostimulants	Variable; not well studied, but anecdotal evidence is strong[79]	Methylphenidate (Ritalin), now in long-acting forms; mocafinil (Provigil) Start at low doses and evaluate for tolerance.
Transcranial magnetic stimulation	Useful noninvasive technique that is increasingly available and effective[80,81]	

Data from Refs.[79-81]

Box 1
Confusion assessment method feature 4: disorganized thinking

Yes/No Questions (See training manual for alternate set of questions)

1. Will a stone float on water?

2. Are there fish in the sea?

3. Does 1 pound weigh more than 2 pounds?

4. Can you use a hammer to pound a nail?

From Ely EW. Confusion Assessment Method for the ICU (CAM-ICU): The Complete Training Manual. Vanderbilt University. Available at: http://www.icudelirium.org/docs/CAM_ICU_training.pdf. Accessed September 19, 2014. Copyright © 2002, E. Wesley Ely, MD, MPH and Vanderbilt University, all rights reserved.

- A well-lit, homelike room, with the dates and clues available (like most skilled nursing facilities do).
- Haloperidol at low doses, starting the 0.25 to 0.5 mg IV or orally. The dose needed to control delirium is almost always less than 3 mg/d.[84]
- Alternatives to haloperidol include quetiapine (Seroquel), risperidone (Risperdal), and olanzapine (Zyprexa).
- If the patient has been on long-term opioids, remember to continue enough to prevent withdrawal.

GASTROINTESTINAL SYMPTOMS
Constipation and Fecal Impaction

Constipation remains a common problem in palliative care no matter what the age, but particularly so in geriatrics. The bowel itself has slower transit, and the list of medications that cause constipation continues to grow. The most common unexpected culprits we see are opioids, ondansetron and similar drugs, and calcium channel blockers.

We have a stepped approach that works for nearly all patients.

1. More fluids, until the urine is light yellow. Do this with all the other remedies.
2. First, we ask "What have you used in the past for constipation?" and start with what the person has used successfully.
3. More dietary fiber, including fruit, fruit juice, bran, supplements. A good recipe is three-quarters of a cup of prune juice, 1 cup of applesauce, and 1 cup of coarse unprocessed wheat bran mix. This can be stored in the refrigerator. Take 1 to 2 large tablespoons, with at least 8 ounces of water. Some add milk of magnesia to the mix for added effect. Do not use bulk-forming agents if the person is dehydrated.
4. Senna tablets. In hospice patients, surfactants such as docusate (Colace) did not add any effect to senna, in a randomized trial.[85] Give enough, until the person has a bowel movement, then continue.
5. Magnesium citrate is inexpensive, readily available, and familiar. We tell people to take about 30 mL (a shot glass) hourly until they have a bowel movement.
6. Generic polyethylene glycol 3350 (Miralax) use has become commonplace and has replaced lactulose, sorbitol, and other osmotic agents.
7. We use subcutaneous methylnaltrexone to reverse the effect of opioids on the bowel,[86] but rarely owing to the success of prevention, and the high cost of the

drug (at least $45/dose.) Do not administer for ileus. There have been a few reports of opioid withdrawal after disruption of the blood–brain barrier by radiation or surgery, so use with caution in patients with recent brain surgery or radiation.

Bowel Obstruction

Bowel obstruction remains a problem in advanced cancer patients, especially rectal, colon, pancreas, and ovarian cancer. It is often associated with carcinomatosis (peritoneal metastases) and malignant ascites, and is strongly associated with a median survival of less than 6 months.[87]

The optimal treatment of malignant bowel obstruction has become less clear-cut in the past years. As Dr von Roenn wrote in 2002, dexamethasone at 4 to 8 mg/d seems to be useful, although there are no randomized trials. Octreotide at standard doses has long been used to reduce small intestinal secretions to levels more manageable by an impaired large intestine, and the preponderance of evidence favors its use.[88] One large, high-power, randomized, controlled trial used all intravenous dexamethasone (8 mg/24 hours), ranitidine (200 mg/24 hours; Zantac), and octreotide (600 μg/ 24 hours by infusion) versus dexamethasone, ranitidine, and placebo. There was no difference in the number of days free of vomiting, the primary endpoint. An adjusted multivariable regression showed more than a 50% reduction in vomiting attributable to octreotide, but with twice the incidence of colicky pain requiring treatment. In addition, octreotide costs at least $15 for each 100-μg dose, typically given 3 times a day, which puts it out of reach of hospice care. The authors concluded that more study was needed.[89]

Nausea and Vomiting

A complete review of nausea and vomiting is beyond the scope of this article, so we have summarized some points we use in our own practice.

- Try to understand the mechanism of the vomiting and nausea. Nausea owing to chemotherapy requires a serotonin or neurokinin-1 blocking drug, whereas nausea owing to constipation or opioids is more likely involving dopamine.
- Vomiting owing to obstruction may or may not have nausea. Antinausea drugs do not help obstruction. Some patients prefer to vomit twice a day rather than have an nasogastric tube.
- Do not use lorazepam (Ativan), diphenhydramine (Benadryl), or haloperidol (ABH) gel for nausea because it is not absorbed[90] and completely ineffective.[91] Up to 60% of hospice patients were given a prescription for ABH or similar gels until recently, with no proof of efficacy; ABH when tested did not work.
- Haloperidol and metoclopramide are the standard drugs we use for both inpatients and outpatients, which is the "Cleveland Clinic" protocol.[92]
- Olanzapine is now generic, $15 for 30 tablets, and is among the best antinausea drugs for chemotherapy-induced nausea[93] and likely for other types of nausea.[94]

SUMMARY

Symptom management continues to improve, but many more improvements are needed. The evidence base behind many of our interventions is based on anecdote.

REFERENCES

1. Brown JA, Von Roenn JH. Symptom management in the older adult [review]. Clin Geriatr Med 2004;20(4):621–40, v–vi.

2. Fisch MJ, Lee JW, Weiss M, et al. Prospective, observational study of pain and analgesic prescribing in medical oncology outpatients with breast, colorectal, lung, or prostate cancer. J Clin Oncol 2012;30(16):1980–8.

3. Okie S. A flood of opioids, a rising tide of deaths. N Engl J Med 2010;363:1981–5.

4. Makris UE, Abrams RC, Gurland B, et al. Management of persistent pain in the older patient: a clinical review. JAMA 2014;312(8):825–36.

5. Drugs.com. Oxycodone prices, coupons and patient assistance programs. Available at: http://www.drugs.com/price-guide/oxycodone#oral-tablet-extended-release-10-mg. Accessed September 19, 2014.

6. Jensen MP. A neuropsychological model of pain: research and clinical implications. J Pain 2010;11(1):2–12.

7. Burakgazi AZ, Messersmith W, Vaidya D, et al. Longitudinal assessment of oxaliplatin-induced neuropathy. Neurology 2011;77(10):980–6.

8. Cruccu G, Sommer C, Anand P, et al. EFNS guidelines on neuropathic pain assessment: revised 2009. Eur J Neurol 2010;17(8):1010–8.

9. Gilron I, Bailey JM, Tu D, et al. Morphine, gabapentin, or their combination for neuropathic pain. N Engl J Med 2005;352(13):1324–34.

10. Gaskell H, Moore RA, Derry S. Oxycodone for neuropathic pain and fibromyalgia in adults. Cochrane Database Syst Rev 2014;(6):CD010692.

11. Pergolizzi J, Böger RH, Budd K, et al. Opioids and the management of chronic severe pain in the elderly: consensus statement of an International Expert Panel with focus on the six clinically most often used World Health Organization Step III opioids (buprenorphine, fentanyl, hydromorphone, methadone, morphine, oxycodone). Pain Pract 2008;8(4):287–313.

12. Bruera E, Palmer JL, Bosnjak S, et al. Methadone versus morphine as a first-line strong opioid for cancer pain: a randomized, double-blind study. J Clin Oncol 2004;22(1):185–92.

13. Moore RA, Wiffen PJ, Derry S, et al. Gabapentin for chronic neuropathic pain and fibromyalgia in adults. Cochrane Database Syst Rev 2014;(4):CD007938.

14. Moulin D, Boulanger A, Clark AJ, et al. Pharmacological management of chronic neuropathic pain: revised consensus statement from the Canadian Pain Society. Pain Res Manag 2014;19(6):328–35.

15. Smith EM, Bakitas MA, Homel P, et al. Preliminary assessment of a neuropathic pain treatment and referral algorithm for patients with cancer. J Pain Symptom Manage 2011;42(6):822–38.

16. Berry JD, Petersen KL. A single dose of gabapentin reduces acute pain and allodynia in patients with herpes zoster. Neurology 2005;65(3):444–7.

17. Jensen-Dahm C, Rowbotham MC, Reda H. Effect of a single dose of pregabalin on herpes zoster pain. Trials 2011;12:55.

18. Johnson RW, Rice AS. Clinical practice. Postherpetic neuralgia. N Engl J Med 2014;371(16):1526–33.

19. Durand JP, Deplanque G, Montheil V, et al. Efficacy of venlafaxine for the prevention and relief of oxaliplatin-induced acute neurotoxicity: results of EFFOX, a randomized, double-blind, placebo-controlled phase III trial. Ann Oncol 2012;23(1):200–5.

20. Smith EM, Pang H, Cirrincione C, et al, Alliance for Clinical Trials in Oncology. Effect of duloxetine on pain, function, and quality of life among patients with chemotherapy-induced painful peripheral neuropathy: a randomized clinical trial. JAMA 2013;309(13):1359–67.

21. Hershman DL, Lacchetti C, Dworkin RH, et al, American Society of Clinical Oncology. Prevention and management of chemotherapy-induced peripheral

neuropathy in survivors of adult cancers: American Society of Clinical Oncology clinical practice guideline. J Clin Oncol 2014;32(18):1941–67.

22. Chochinov HM, Wilson KG, Enns M, et al. "Are you depressed?" Screening for depression in the terminally ill. Am J Psychiatry 1997;154(5):674–6.

23. Zimmerman M, Ruggero CJ, Chelminski I, et al. Developing brief scales for use in clinical practice: the reliability and validity of single-item self-report measures of depression symptom severity, psychosocial impairment due to depression, and quality of life. J Clin Psychiatry 2006;67(10):1536–41.

24. Hughes EF, Wu AW, Carducci MA, et al. What can I do? Recommendations for responding to issues identified by patient-reported outcomes assessments used in clinical practice [review]. J Support Oncol 2012;10(4):143–8.

25. Hurlow A, Bennett MI, Robb KA, et al. Transcutaneous electric nerve stimulation (TENS) for cancer pain in adults [review]. Cochrane Database Syst Rev 2012;(3):CD006276.

26. Colvin LA, Johnson PR, Mitchell R, et al. From bench to bedside: a case of rapid reversal of bortezomib-induced neuropathic pain by the TRPM8 activator, menthol. J Clin Oncol 2008;26(27):4519–20.

27. Smith TJ, Coyne PJ, Parker GL, et al. Pilot trial of a patient-specific cutaneous electrostimulation device (MC5-A Calmare®) for chemotherapy-induced peripheral neuropathy. J Pain Symptom Manage 2010;40(6):883–91.

28. Pachman DR, Weisbrod BL, Seisler DK, et al. Pilot evaluation of Scrambler therapy for the treatment of chemotherapy-induced peripheral neuropathy. Support Care Cancer 2014. [Epub ahead of print].

29. Smith TJ, Marineo G. Treatment of postherpetic pain with scrambler therapy, a patient-specific neurocutaneous electrical stimulation device. Am J Hosp Palliat Care 2013. [Epub ahead of print].

30. Guiseppe M, Vittorio I, Cristiano G, et al. MC5-A scrambler therapy relieves chronic neuropathic pain more effectively than guideline based drug management. J Pain Symptom Manage 2012;43(1):87–95.

31. Swislocki A, Orth M, Bales M, et al. A randomized clinical trial of the effectiveness of photon stimulation on pain, sensation, and quality of life in patients with diabetic peripheral neuropathy. J Pain Symptom Manage 2010;39(1):88–99.

32. Heiskanen T, Mätzke S, Haakana S, et al. Transdermal fentanyl in cachectic cancer patients. Pain 2009;144(1–2):218–22.

33. Prommer EE. Tramadol: does it have a role in cancer pain management? J Opioid Manag 2005;1(3):131–8.

34. Arbaiza D, Vidal O. Tramadol in the treatment of neuropathic cancer pain: a double-blind, placebo-controlled study. Clin Drug Investig 2007;27(1):75–83.

35. Candiotti KA, Gitlin MC. Review of the effect of opioid-related side effects on the undertreatment of moderate to severe chronic non-cancer pain: tapentadol, a step toward a solution? Curr Med Res Opin 2010;26(7):1677–84.

36. Wilcock A, Beattie JM. Prolonged QT interval and methadone: implications for palliative care. Curr Opin Support Palliat Care 2009;3(4):252–7.

37. Derry S, Moore RA, Rabbie R. Topical NSAIDs for chronic musculoskeletal pain in adults. Cochrane Database Syst Rev 2012;(9):CD007400.

38. Lin YC, Kuan TS, Hsieh PC, et al. Therapeutic effects of lidocaine patch on myofascial pain syndrome of the upper trapezius: a randomized, double-blind, placebo-controlled study. Am J Phys Med Rehabil 2012;91(10):871–82.

39. Patrick DL, Cleeland CS, von Moos R, et al. Pain outcomes in patients with bone metastases from advanced cancer: assessment and management with bone-targeting agents. Support Care Cancer 2014. [Epub ahead of print].

40. Scott LJ, Muir VJ. Denosumab: in the prevention of skeletal-related events in patients with bone metastases from solid tumours. Drugs 2011;71(8):1059–69.
41. Coleman R, Body JJ, Aapro M, et al, ESMO Guidelines Working Group. Bone health in cancer patients: ESMO Clinical Practice Guidelines. Ann Oncol 2014; 25(Suppl 3):iii124–37.
42. Schuster JM, Smith TJ, Coyne PJ, et al. Clinic offering affordable radiation therapy to increase access to care for patients enrolled in hospice. J Oncol Pract 2014;10(6):e390–5.
43. Mercadante S, Villari P, Ferrera P, et al. Optimization of opioid therapy for preventing incident pain associated with bone metastases. J Pain Symptom Manage 2004;28(5):505–10.
44. Mercadante S, Villari P, Ferrera P, et al. Opioid switching and burst ketamine to improve the opioid response in patients with movement-related pain due to bone metastases. Clin J Pain 2009;25(7):648–9.
45. Mercadante S, Villari P, Ferrera P. Pamidronate in incident pain due to bone metastases. J Pain Symptom Manage 2001;22(2):630–1.
46. Xander C, Meerpohl JJ, Galandi D, et al. Pharmacological interventions for pruritus in adult palliative care patients. Cochrane Database Syst Rev 2013;6: CD008320.
47. Siemens W, Xander C, Meerpohl JJ, et al. Drug treatments for pruritus in adult palliative care. Dtsch Arztebl Int 2014;111(50):863–70.
48. Unotoro J, Nonaka E, Takita N, et al. Paroxetine treatment of 3 cases of cholestatic pruritus due to gastrointestinal malignancy. Nihon Shokakibyo Gakkai Zasshi 2010;107(2):257–62 [Japanese].
49. Mayo MJ, Handem I, Saldana S, et al. Sertraline as a first-line treatment for cholestatic pruritus. Hepatology 2007;45(3):666–74.
50. Ryan NM, Birring SS, Gibson PG. Gabapentin for refractory chronic cough: a randomised, double-blind, placebo-controlled trial. Lancet 2012;380(9853):1583–9.
51. Ryan NM. A review on the efficacy and safety of gabapentin in the treatment of chronic cough. Expert Opin Pharmacother 2015;16(1):135–45.
52. Barton DL, Liu H, Dakhil SR, et al. Wisconsin Ginseng (Panax quinquefolius) to improve cancer-related fatigue: a randomized, double-blind trial, N07C2. J Natl Cancer Inst 2013;105(16):1230–8.
53. Yennurajalingam S, Frisbee-Hume S, Palmer JL, et al. Reduction of cancer-related fatigue with dexamethasone: a double-blind, randomized, placebo-controlled trial in patients with advanced cancer. J Clin Oncol 2013;31(25):3076–82.
54. Bruera E, Driver L, Barnes EA, et al. Patient-controlled methylphenidate for the management of fatigue in patients with advanced cancer: a preliminary report. J Clin Oncol 2003;21(23):4439–43.
55. Bruera E, Valero V, Driver L, et al. Patient-controlled methylphenidate for cancer fatigue: a double-blind, randomized, placebo-controlled trial. J Clin Oncol 2006; 24(13):2073–8.
56. Moraska AR, Sood A, Dakhil SR, et al. Phase III, randomized, double-blind, placebo-controlled study of long-acting methylphenidate for cancer-related fatigue: North Central Cancer Treatment Group NCCTG-N05C7 trial. J Clin Oncol 2010; 28(23):3673–9.
57. Spathis A, Fife K, Blackhall F, et al. Modafinil for the treatment of fatigue in lung cancer: results of a placebo-controlled, double-blind, randomized trial. J Clin Oncol 2014;32(18):1882–8.
58. Breitbart W, Alici Y. Psychostimulants for cancer-related fatigue [review]. J Natl Compr Canc Netw 2010;8(8):933–42.

59. Yennurajalingam S, Palmer JL, Chacko R, et al. Factors associated with response to methylphenidate in advanced cancer patients. Oncologist 2011;16(2):246–53.

60. Lynn J, Teno JM, Phillips RS, et al. Perceptions by family members of the dying experience of older and seriously ill patients. SUPPORT Investigators. Study to Understand Prognoses and Preferences for Outcomes and Risks of Treatments. Ann Intern Med 1997;126(2):97–106.

61. Uronis HE, Currow DC, McCrory DC, et al. Oxygen for relief of dyspnoea in mildly- or non-hypoxaemic patients with cancer: a systematic review and meta-analysis. Br J Cancer 2008;98(2):294–9.

62. Abernethy AP, McDonald CF, Frith PA, et al. Effect of palliative oxygen versus room air in relief of breathlessness in patients with refractory dyspnoea: a double-blind, randomised controlled trial. Lancet 2010;376(9743):784–93.

63. Uronis H, McCrory DC, Samsa G, et al. Symptomatic oxygen for non-hypoxaemic chronic obstructive pulmonary disease [review]. Cochrane Database Syst Rev 2011;(6):CD006429.

64. Ameer F, Carson KV, Usmani ZA, et al. Ambulatory oxygen for people with chronic obstructive pulmonary disease who are not hypoxaemic at rest. Cochrane Database Syst Rev 2014;(6):CD000238.

65. Varkey B. Opioids for palliation of refractory dyspnea in chronic obstructive pulmonary disease patients. Curr Opin Pulm Med 2010;16(2):150–4.

66. Johnson MJ, Hui D, Currow DC. Opioids, exertion, and dyspnea: a review of the evidence. Am J Hosp Palliat Care 2014 [pii:1049909114552692]. [Epub ahead of print].

67. Gifford AH, Mahler DA, Waterman LA, et al. Neuromodulatory effect of endogenous opioids on the intensity and unpleasantness of breathlessness during resistive load breathing in COPD. COPD 2011;8(3):160–6.

68. Currow DC, McDonald C, Oaten S, et al. Once-daily opioids for chronic dyspnea: a dose increment and pharmacovigilance study. J Pain Symptom Manage 2011; 42(3):388–99.

69. Allcroft P, Margitanovic V, Greene A, et al. The role of benzodiazepines in breathlessness: a single site, open label pilot of sustained release morphine together with clonazepam. J Palliat Med 2013;16(7):741–4.

70. Simon ST, Niemand AM, Benalia H, et al. Acceptability and preferences of six different routes of drug application for acute breathlessness: a comparison study between the United Kingdom and Germany. J Palliat Med 2012;15(12):1374–81.

71. Marciniuk D, Goodridge D, Hernandez P, et al. Managing dyspnea in patients with advanced chronic obstructive pulmonary disease: a Canadian Thoracic Society clinical practice guideline. Can Respir J 2011;18(2):69–78.

72. Coyne P, Ramakrishnan V, Smith TJ. Nebulized fentanyl improves patients' perception of breathing, respiratory rate, and oxygen saturation in dyspnea. J Pain Symptom Manage 2002;23:157–60.

73. Smith TJ, Coyne P, French W, et al. Failure to accrue to a study of nebulized fentanyl for dyspnea: lessons learned. J Palliat Med 2009;12(9):771–2.

74. Hirsch CA, Marriott JF, Faull CM. Influences on the decision to prescribe or administer anticholinergic drugs to treat death rattle: a focus group study. Palliat Med 2013;27(8):732–8.

75. Mercadamte S. Death rattle: critical review and research agenda. Support Care Cancer 2014;22(2):571–5.

76. Lokker ME, van Zuylen L, van der Rijt CC, et al. Prevalence, impact, and treatment of death rattle: a systematic review. J Pain Symptom Manage 2014;47(1): 105–22.

77. Flicker C, Ferris SH, Serby M. Hypersensitivity to scopolamine in the elderly. Psychopharmacology (Berl) 1992;107(2–3):437–41.
78. Twomey S, Dowling M. Management of death rattle at end of life. Br J Nurs 2013; 22(2):81–5.
79. Hardy SE. Methylphenidate for the treatment of depressive symptoms, including fatigue and apathy, in medically ill older adults and terminally ill adults. Am J Geriatr Pharmacother 2009;7(1):34–59.
80. Transcranial Magnetic Stimulation for the Treatment of Adults with PTSD, GAD, or Depression: A Review of Clinical Effectiveness and Guidelines [Internet]. CADTH Rapid Response Reports. Ottawa (ON): Canadian Agency for Drugs and Technologies in Health; 2014.
81. Allan CL, Herrmann LL, Ebmeier KP. Transcranial magnetic stimulation in the management of mood disorders. Neuropsychobiology 2011;64(3):163–9.
82. Inouye SK, van Dyck CH, Alessi CA, et al. Clarifying confusion: the confusion assessment method. A new method for detection of delirium. Ann Intern Med 1990;113(12):941–8.
83. Available at: http://www.eperc.mcw.edu/EPERC/FastFactsIndex/ff_125.htm. Accessed September 19, 2014.
84. Hui D, Bush SH, Gallo LE, et al. Neuroleptic dose in the management of delirium in patients with advanced cancer. J Pain Symptom Manage 2010;39(2):186–96.
85. Tarumi Y, Wilson MP, Szafran O, et al. Randomized, double-blind, placebo-controlled trial of oral docusate in the management of constipation in hospice patients. J Pain Symptom Manage 2013;45(1):2–13.
86. Thomas J, Karver S, Cooney GA, et al. Methylnaltrexone for opioid-induced constipation in advanced illness. N Engl J Med 2008;358(22):2332–43.
87. Salpeter SR, Malter DS, Luo EJ, et al. Systematic review of cancer presentations with a median survival of six months or less [review]. J Palliat Med 2012;15(2): 175–85.
88. Mercadante S, Porzio G. Octreotide for malignant bowel obstruction: twenty years after. Crit Rev Oncol Hematol 2012;83(3):388–92.
89. Currow DC, Quinn S, Agar M, et al. Double-blind, placebo-controlled, randomized trial of octreotide in malignant bowel obstruction. J Pain Symptom Manage 2014. http://dx.doi.org/10.1016/j.jpainsymman.2014.09.013.
90. Smith TJ, Ritter JK, Poklis JL, et al. ABH gel is not absorbed from the skin of normal volunteers. J Pain Symptom Manage 2012;43(5):961–6.
91. Fletcher DS, Coyne PJ, Dodson PW, et al. A randomized trial of the effectiveness of topical "ABH Gel" (Ativan(®), Benadryl(®), Haldol(®)) vs. placebo in cancer patients with nausea. J Pain Symptom Manage 2014;48(5):797–803.
92. Gupta M, Davis M, LeGrand S, et al. Nausea and vomiting in advanced cancer: the Cleveland Clinic protocol. J Support Oncol 2013;11(1):8–13.
93. Hocking CM, Kichenadasse G. Olanzapine for chemotherapy-induced nausea and vomiting: a systematic review [review]. Support Care Cancer 2014;22(4): 1143–51.
94. Prommer E. Olanzapine: palliative medicine update [review]. Am J Hosp Palliat Care 2013;30(1):75–82.

Complementary and Integrative Medicine for Older Adults in Palliative Care

Madeline Leong, MD[a,*], Thomas J. Smith, MD[a],
Anastasia Rowland-Seymour, MD[b]

KEYWORDS

- Integrative medicine • Complementary medicine • Alternative medicine
- Palliative care

KEY POINTS

- Complementary and Integrative Medicine can benefit patients in palliative care.
- Clinicians should ask patients about their use of complementary and alternative therapies.
- When prescribing natural products, clinicians should consider any natural product-drug interactions, patient comorbidities, and the quality or brand of the natural product.

INTRODUCTION
What is Complementary and Integrative Medicine?

Complementary and Integrative Medicine (CIM) refers to the use of nonmainstream therapies along with conventional treatment.[1] The Arizona Center for Integrative Medicine defines CIM as "healing-oriented medicine that … emphasizes the therapeutic relationship between practitioner and patient, is informed by evidence, and makes use of all appropriate therapies."[2] Although "complementary medicine" and "integrative medicine" have been used interchangeably, the term "alternative medicine" indicates the use of a nonmainstream approach in place of conventional medicine.[1] Most nonconventional medicine modalities that are used in the United States are those used in addition to conventional medicine.[3] In this article, the focus is on safe, effective CIM for older adults who require palliative care.

CIM is broad and encompasses diverse therapies. According to the National Center for Complementary and Integrative Health (NCCIH), 3 main categories of CIM are (1) natural products, (2) mind and body practices, and (3) other complementary health approaches.[1]

The authors have no conflict of interest.
[a] Department of Palliative Care, Johns Hopkins Hospital, 600 North Wolfe Street, Blalock 369, Baltimore, MD 21287, USA; [b] Program in Integrative Medicine, Division of General Internal Medicine, Johns Hopkins Hospital, 600 North Wolfe Street, Baltimore, MD 21287, USA
* Corresponding author.
E-mail address: mkunsbe1@jhmi.edu

Natural products (ie, supplements) include herbs, botanicals, vitamins, minerals, probiotics, and other substances derived from natural sources. Examples of mind and body practices are acupuncture, massage, mediation, movement therapies, relaxation techniques, spinal manipulation, tai chi, qi gong, and yoga. Other complementary health approaches include Ayurvedic medicine, traditional Chinese medicine, homeopathy, and naturopathy.

Herein, natural products and mind and body practices are highlighted; an in-depth analysis of traditional Chinese medicine or Ayurvedic medicine is beyond the scope this article.

In addition to being widely varied, CIM is extremely common, with 38.3% of the US population using complementary medicine modalities in 2007.[4] CIM is similarly prevalent in older adults. In a study of 1445 Mexican Americans aged 65 or older, 31.6% used nonmainstream therapies.[5] In a study of 95 African Americans aged 60 or older, 88.4% reported use of nonmainstream therapies in the past year.[6] Overall, approximately 15% to 40% of older adults are thought to use nonmainstream therapies.[7] Because these therapies can significantly impact health, especially in frail older adults, it is important to ask patients about their use.

Ask About Integrative Medicine

Although patients frequently use nonmainstream therapies, they may not actively disclose this information. In a recent survey of 1013 adults aged 50 or older, 67% had not discussed their use of nonmainstream therapies with a clinician.[8] The primary reason for this (42%) was that the clinician never asked.

To encourage patients and physicians to discuss nonmainstream therapies, NCCIH created a public health campaign in 2008: *Time to Talk* provides resources for patients, clinicians, and community organizations.[9] Various authors have proposed different ways to ask about nonmainstream therapies. One may ask, "Have you used any of the following types of complementary or alternative medicine in the past year: herbal products or dietary supplements, massage therapy or chiropractic manipulation, mind-body practices, or naturopathy?"[8] A simpler alternative is to ask: "Are you doing anything else for this condition?"[10]

RECOMMENDATIONS FOR SPECIFIC SYMPTOMS

CIM can provide significant benefits for patients requiring palliative care. However, because of the immense scope of CIM, it is difficult to provide a discussion of every possible interaction between CIM and palliative care. Therefore, in this article, the focus is on the use of CIM to ameliorate physical symptoms in palliative care patients. Symptoms were selected based on the Memorial Symptom Assessment Scale, an instrument frequently used in palliative care. However, this article will not address depression, anxiety, or memory/concentration because these subjects are too broad for this review.

The following symptoms are reviewed: pain, nausea, fatigue, constipation, and diarrhea. Also included are brief recommendations for cough, dry mouth, pruritus, and anorexia.

Pain

Scenario 1

A 75-year-old man has a past medical history of Hepatitis C, peptic ulcer disease, and osteoarthritis. He complains of chronic bilateral knee pain. He takes 22 medications a day and has been counseled about polypharmacy. He asks for a "safe and natural" medication for his pain. What do you recommend?

Complementary approaches to pain management include massage, acupuncture, and herbal supplements. Low-risk solutions to pain are even more important in an elderly population because the clinician must consider polypharmacy, altered metabolism of medications, and increased neuropsychiatric sensitivity to medications.

Massage has been used for pain management in many disorders with varying results.[11] Massage has been shown to improve functional status in conditions such as neck pain[12] and quality-of-life measures in patients with end-stage cancer.[13]

Acupuncture offers another nonpharmacologic approach to pain management. Evidence suggests that acupuncture may be useful for acute pain or postoperative pain.[14–16] There are conflicting data on the use of acupuncture for osteoarthritis, particularly chronic knee pain.[17,18] Other studies show modest positive findings for the use of acupuncture in some chronic pain syndromes[19,20] but not in fibromyalgia.[21]

The potential serious adverse event of a pneumothorax due to acupuncture is often cited, yet in the authors' experience this happens rarely. Analysis of a cohort in which acupuncture is used by most of the population may provide some indication of the prevalence of this adverse event. A recent study indicates that 1100 acupuncture-related adverse events were reported in the Republic of Korea between 1999 and 2010.[22] Unfortunately, with this data alone, there is no way to calculate the risk of injury from acupuncture. A very conservative estimate, assuming 35% of Korean citizens used acupuncture at least once annually, provides an adverse event rate of 0.0005%.

In addition to massage and acupuncture, herbal supplements are often used as adjuvants for pain management. Supplements commonly recommended for pain are Turmeric (Curcumin) and ginger.

Curcumin has been used for acute pain in the postsurgical setting[23] and for chronic pain (eg, in osteoarthritis and neuropathy).[24,25] When compared with standard nonsteroidal anti-inflammatory drug (NSAID) use in the treatment of knee osteoarthritis, Curcumin was equally effective (ibuprofen 1200 mg/d vs *Curcuma domestica* extracts 1500 mg/d for 4 weeks).[26] Curcumin may be used as an adjuvant to standard NSAID use and may allow for decreased total NSAID use, thereby reducing the risk of NSAID-related adverse events.[24] Its mode of action is thought to be through blockade of prostaglandin PGE_2 production.[27] Although Curcumin acts through an anti-inflammatory mechanism similar to that of the COX-2 inhibitors, it seems to have fewer gastrointestinal (GI) adverse effects, perhaps because of histamine blocking effects.[28] Moreover, Curcumin alleviates dyspepsia in adults.[29] Animal data suggest that Curcumin may even be gastroprotective when administered 30 minutes before indomethacin.[30]

As an analgesic, ginger has a mode of action similar to that of Curcumin.[31] Although the data for ginger as an analgesic are not as robust as the data for Curcumin,[32] ginger has been shown to be effective for knee osteoarthritis.[33–35] Ginger and Curcumin have been combined in multiple proprietary preparations for improved pain relief, and there are data to suggest the effectiveness of this combination therapy.[36,37] Similarly, ginger has been combined with other herbs to create various useful analgesic products.[38]

In **Scenario 1**, the clinician could recommend: (1) *C domestica* extracts 1500 mg daily or (2) Ginger extract (Zintona EC) 250 mg 4 times daily.[35]

Nausea

Scenario 2

A 65-year-old woman is diagnosed with metastatic pancreatic cancer. She is from India and has a strong interest in Ayurveda and CIM. She plans to start chemotherapy but is concerned about adverse effects, especially nausea and vomiting. What do you recommend?

Nausea is a frequent complaint associated with cancer and its related therapies. The most promising complementary therapies for nausea are ginger, acupuncture, and acupressure.

Ginger has been used for nausea in a myriad of instances, including postoperative nausea,[39] HIV/antiretroviral-induced nausea,[40] and pregnancy-associated nausea.[41,42] Ginger may decrease chemotherapy-related nausea; however, the data are conflicting.[43,44] For this reason, a more definitive trial is underway.[45]

Acupuncture has also been used for chemotherapy-related nausea, but again, studies show mixed results.[46,47] The use of acupressure, in the form of a wristband, popularly found under the brand name "Sea-Band", has been used for chemotherapy-related nausea with good effect.[48–50] Acupressure was additionally noted to be effective for migraine-related nausea[51] but not for postoperative nausea.[52,53]

In **Scenario 2**, the clinician could recommend (1) powdered ginger root 1 g daily[54] or (2) acupressure with a Sea-Band.

Fatigue

Fatigue has many potential causes, such as insomnia, chemotherapy, and depression.

Insomnia

Insomnia is a common cause of fatigue in the elderly. Therapies for insomnia include magnesium, melatonin, and acupuncture.

Magnesium is often used as a muscle relaxant and an anxiolytic agent; as such, it can be useful for treating insomnia.[55–57] Individuals with primary insomnia have decreased melatonin levels.[58] One study showed a correlation between magnesium supplementation and increased melatonin secretion levels.[59] Based on this data, magnesium may be used to treat primary insomnia in the elderly (dose: elemental magnesium 300 mg nightly or magnesium oxide 500 mg nightly).

In conditions with a delayed sleep phase, melatonin improves circadian rhythm sleep disturbances. In fact, melatonin has orphan drug status for this indication in the blind population.[60] For individuals with decreased melatonin levels and primary insomnia, adding melatonin modestly decreases sleep latency (time to sleep). Melatonin is most effective in the elderly, who have lower levels of endogenous melatonin.[61–63] It seems to be more useful in elderly women than in elderly men, presumably because of lower melatonin levels in women.[64]

In younger populations, the herb valerian root extract may be used as an anxiolytic, sedative, and hypnotic.[65] Valerian, however, affects the metabolism of many psychotropic medications through the CYP 450 2D6 mechanism[66] and the metabolism of several chemotherapeutic agents through CYP 450 3A4.[67] Therefore, it is not recommended for elderly patients in palliative care.

Finally, acupuncture has been used with mixed results for insomnia.[68–71]

Cancer-related fatigue

Cancer-related fatigue is a major cause of disability in the palliative care population. Ginseng may improve fatigue in patients undergoing cancer-related therapies.[72–74] It is important to note that the type of ginseng studied was *Panax quinquefolius* (American ginseng) at doses of 1000–2000 mg daily.[75]

Studies also suggest that acupuncture benefits patients with cancer-related fatigue.[73,76,77] However, the results are not conclusive because of the studies' methodological limitations.[77,78]

Constipation

Constipation increases with age for many reasons, including physiologic changes, medication effects, dietary factors, and activity levels. Opioids are a major cause of constipation in the palliative care population. In the general population, the mainstay of constipation treatment is dietary changes (eg, increased fiber intake). However, for the palliative care population, this approach is insufficient due to narcotic use and may even be contraindicated in patients who cannot comply with large-volume fluid consumption.

Complementary therapies for constipation are magnesium, Triphala, Senna, clinical hypnosis, and probiotics. It is important to note that many constipation regimens used in the elderly have been predominantly studied in nonpalliative care settings.[79]

Magnesium is often used as part of a bowel preparation in the form of magnesium citrate. There are also some data that suggest it may prevent constipation in patients using opiates.[80]

Triphala, an Ayurvedic herb combination of "3 fruits" (Indian Gooseberry, *Terminalia belerica*, and *Terminalia chebula*), has been used to treat constipation-predominant irritable bowel syndrome. However, there is only one readily available research study on its use for constipation in the elderly.[81] As Triphala is thought to act similarly to soluble fiber, further studies are needed to ensure its safety in a palliative care population.

Senna (from the plant *Senna alexandrina*) has been effective for constipation in patients with cancer.[82,83] In the past, clinicians discouraged long-term Senna use for fear of increased dependence and potential alteration of GI motility. Now studies indicate that long-term Senna use is not associated with increased GI tumors, nor is it associated with alteration of enteric nerves or visceral smooth muscle function. Therefore, Senna is thought to be safe for chronic use.[84,85]

Clinical hypnosis (Palsson protocol) effectively treats constipation in constipation-predominant irritable bowel syndrome.[86,87] To the authors' knowledge, however, there are no data on the use of clinical hypnosis for constipation in the palliative care population.

In functional constipation syndromes, probiotics may improve intestinal transit time, stool frequency, and stool consistency.[88] In the elderly population, probiotics may have unique health benefits because they maintain GI flora, improve colonization resistance, and prevent diarrhea syndromes.[89]

However, a theoretic concern remains: Are probiotics safe for the immunocompromised or do they pose an increased risk of sepsis?[90] There have been case reports of fungemia associated with probiotic administration.[91] However, a recent systematic review[92] indicates probiotics are well-tolerated, even among immunocompromised patients. Many of the studies included in the systematic review lacked sufficient detail on adverse events. Because of the limited data, it is recommended that immunocompromised patients avoid probiotics.

Diarrhea

For diarrhea, the standard BRAT diet (bananas, rice, apples, tea and toast) continues to be effective. Banana flakes have been shown to control diarrhea in critically ill enterally fed patients.[93] Banana flakes are often hard to find in the hospital setting; however, they are marketed as a medical agent under the name Kanana Banana.

Cough, Dry Mouth, Pruritus, and Anorexia

The following symptoms of cough, dry mouth, pruritus, and anorexia have been frequently managed with supplements. However, there are few studies to substantiate the use of nonconventional remedies. **Tables 1** and **2** offer potential therapies and doses that can be used. Drug-herb interactions can be researched using a reputable

Table 1
Therapies for cough

Type	Therapy	Dosage
Associated with pharyngitis/sore throat	Hyssop	• Two 445-mg capsules 3 times a day • 10–15 drops of hyssop extract (12%–14% by volume) in water 2 or 3 times a day
	Honey	• 2.5–10 mL (0.5–2 teaspoons) every night at bedtime
Due to upper airway cough syndrome (formerly known as postnasal drip)	Marshmallow root	• Dried leaf 2–5 g 3 times a day • Dried root 5 g 3 times a day • Liquid leaf/root extract (1:1 in 25% alcohol) 2–5 mL 3 times a day • Root syrup 2–10 mL tid when necessary
Associated with gastroesophageal reflux disease	Licorice	No standard dosage

Data from Natural Medicines Comprehensive Database. Available at: www.naturaldatabase.com. Accessed December 01, 2014.

secondary source such as Natural Standard[94] or Natural Medicine Comprehensive Database.[95]

INTEGRATIVE MEDICINE AND GERIATRICS: KEY CONSIDERATIONS

Use of CIM in a geriatric population poses unique challenges as does the use of CIM in the terminally ill. There is little research to guide clinical practice in these areas. The authors recommend the following strategies, based on expert opinion.

In Patients with Limited Renal or Hepatic Function, Avoid Natural Products

With limited hepatic or renal clearance, the potential for natural product-drug interactions is immense. For example, some herbs, such as Licorice root, cause hyperkalemia, which can be dangerous in a patient on hemodialysis.[97] For patients with decreased renal or hepatic function, it is recommended to explain that natural products pose a high risk of adverse effects.

As a side note, herbs that cause hepatotoxicity should be avoided in all cases (**Table 3**).

Table 2
Therapies for dry mouth, pruritis, and anorexia

Symptom	Therapy	Dosage
Dry mouth	Biotene[96]	• Available as toothpaste, mouthwash, and chewing gum
Pruritus (Itching)	Topical camphor	• 3%–11% ointment 2 times a day when necessary
Anorexia	Branched-chain amino acids	• Granules of valine, leucine, and isoleucine 4 g 3 times a day
	Cannabis (Dronabinol)	• 2.5–10 mg 2 times a day

Data from Warde P, Kroll B, O'Sullivan B, et al. A phase II study of Biotene in the treatment of post-radiation xerostomia in patients with head and neck cancer. Support Care Cancer 2000;8(3):203–8; and Natural Medicines Comprehensive Database. Available at: www.naturaldatabase.com. Accessed December 01, 2014.

Table 3
Worrisome herbs

Name	Purported Uses	Possible Dangers	Comments
Aconite (aconiti tuber, conitum, radix aconiti)	Inflammation, joint pain, wounds, gout	Toxicity, nausea, vomiting, low blood pressure, respiratory-system paralysis, heart-rhythm disorders, death	Unsafe. Aconite is the most common cause of severe herbal poisoning in Hong Kong
Bitter orange (aurantii fructus, Citrus aurantium, zhi shi)	Weight loss, nasal congestion, allergies	Fainting, heart-rhythm disorders, heart attack, stroke, death	Possibly unsafe. Contains synephrine, which is similar to ephedrine, banned by the FDA in 2004. Risks might be higher when taken with herbs that contain caffeine.
Chaparral (creosote bush, Larrea divaricata, larreastat)	Colds, weight loss, infections, inflammation, cancer, detoxification	Liver damage, kidney problems	Likely unsafe. The FDA advises people not to take chaparral.
Colloidal silver (ionic silver, native silver, silver in suspending agent)	Fungal and other infections, Lyme disease, rosacea, psoriasis, food poisoning, chronic fatigue syndrome, HIV/AIDS	Bluish skin, mucous membrane discoloration, neurologic problems, kidney damage	Likely unsafe. The FDA advised consumers about the risk of discoloration on October 6, 2009.
Coltsfoot (coughwort, farfarae folium leaf, foalswort)	Cough, sore throat, laryngitis, bronchitis, asthma	Liver damage, cancer	Likely unsafe
Comfrey (blackwort, common comfrey, slippery root)	Cough, heavy menstrual periods, chest pain, cancer	Liver damage, cancer	Likely unsafe. The FDA advised manufacturers to remove comfrey products from the market in July 2001.

(continued on next page)

Table 3
(continued)

Name	Purported Uses	Possible Dangers	Comments
Country mallow (heartleaf, Sida cordifolia, silky white mallow)	Nasal congestion, allergies, asthma, weight loss, bronchitis	Heart attack, heart arrhythmia, stroke, death	Likely unsafe. Possible dangers linked with its ephedrine alkaloids, banned by the FDA in 2004.
Germanium (Ge, Ge-132, germanium-132)	Pain, infections, glaucoma, liver problems, arthritis, osteoporosis, heart disease, HIV/AIDS, cancer	Kidney damage, death	Likely unsafe. The FDA warned in 1993 that it was linked to serious adverse events.
Greater celandine (celandine, chelidonii herba, Chelidonium majus)	Upset stomach, irritable bowel syndrome, liver disorders, detoxification, cancer	Liver damage	Possibly unsafe
Kava (awa, Piper methysticum, kava-kava)	Anxiety (possibly effective)	Liver damage	Possibly unsafe. The FDA issued a warning to consumers in March 2002. Banned in Germany, Canada, and Switzerland.
Lobelia (asthma weed, Lobelia inflata, pukeweed, vomit wort)	Coughing, bronchitis, asthma, smoking cessation (possibly ineffective)	Toxicity; overdose can cause fast heartbeat, very low blood pressure, coma, possibly death	Likely unsafe. The FDA warned in 1993 that it was linked to serious adverse events.
Yohimbe (yohimbine, Corynanthe yohimbi, Corynanthe johimbi)	Aphrodisiac, chest pain, diabetic complications, depression; erectile dysfunction (possibly effective)	Usual doses can cause high blood pressure, rapid heart rate; high doses can cause severe low blood pressure, heart problems, death	Possibly unsafe for use without medical supervision because it contains a prescription drug, yohimbine. The FDA warned in 1993 that reports of serious adverse events were under investigation.

Abbreviation: FDA, US Food and Drug Administration.
Data from Natural Medicines Comprehensive Database. 2014. Available at: http://naturaldatabase.therapeuticresearch.com. Accessed December 01, 2014.

Check for Natural Product-Drug Interactions

Natural products may interact with prescription drugs, especially in the setting of polypharmacy. One study observed 171 adults (average age 57.1) who used natural products. Of these, 45.2% were at risk for potentially severe natural product-drug interactions.[98]

With this in mind, the clinician may use several databases to check for natural product-drug interactions. For example, the Natural Medicines Comprehensive Database[95] provides an online "Natural Product/Drug Interaction Checker." Another alternative is pharmacy consultation.

Advise Patients to Obtain High-Quality Natural Products

Unlike manufacturers of pharmaceuticals, manufacturers of natural products are not required to submit rigorous evidence of safety before marketing. Because of this, natural products may be of poor quality or contain harmful ingredients. According to the Drug-Induced Liver Injury Network, 130 cases of liver injury likely due to natural products were reported between 2004 and 2013.[99] The clinician should caution patients about the dangers of some untested natural products.

To identify high-quality natural products, the authors suggest reading labels: a high-quality natural product is often labeled "NSF" (certified by the National Sanitation Foundation)[100] or "USP" (certified by the United States Pharmacopeial Convention).[101] A less reliable notation is "GMP", which indicates that the product was created under Good Manufacturing Practices.

Educational Resources

The following Web sites provide useful information about CIM:

- NCCIH (https://nccih.nih.gov/news/camstats/2007)
- Consumer Lab: independent testing of health and nutritional products (www.consumerlab.com)
- Natural Medicines Comprehensive Database (http://naturaldatabase.therapeutic research.com/)

SUMMARY

CIM offers many benefits to patients in palliative care. CIM is widespread, and clinicians should ask patients about their use of complementary and alternative therapies. Many complementary therapies are available for common symptoms, including pain, nausea, fatigue, and constipation.

When recommending natural products for a palliative care population, the clinician should be aware of the following caveats:

1. The potential harm of natural products in patients with limited renal or hepatic function
2. The potential harm of natural product-drug interactions
3. The potential harm of natural products due to poor manufacturing quality.

In addition to natural products, the clinician should consider mind and body practices and other complementary health approaches, such as acupuncture and massage. Because there are relatively few studies of CIM in the palliative care population, further research is needed to guide care.

REFERENCES

1. Complementary, alternative, or integrative health: what's in a name? 2008. Available at: http://nccam.nih.gov/health/whatiscam. Accessed December 01, 2014.

2. What is Integrative Medicine? 2014. Available at: http://integrativemedicine. arizona.edu/about/definition.html. Accessed December 01, 2014.

3. Astin JA. Why patients use alternative medicine: results of a national study. JAMA 1998;279(19):1548–53.

4. 2007 Statistics on CAM Use in the United States. 2013. Available at: http:// nccam.nih.gov/news/camstats/2007. Accessed December 01, 2014.

5. Loera JA, Reyes-Ortiz C, Kuo YF. Predictors of complementary and alternative medicine use among older Mexican Americans. Complement Ther Clin Pract 2007;13(4):224–31.

6. Ryder PT, Wolpert B, Orwig D, et al. Complementary and alternative medicine use among older urban African Americans: individual and neighborhood associations. J Natl Med Assoc 2008;100(10):1186–92.

7. Sternberg SA, Chandran A, Sikka M. Alternative therapy use by elderly African Americans attending a community clinic. J Am Geriatr Soc 2003;51(12): 1768–72.

8. AARP and National Center for Complementary and Alternative Medicine Survey Report. 2011.

9. Time to Talk. 2008. Available at: https://nccih.nih.gov/timetotalk. Accessed December 01, 2014.

10. Steyer TE. Complementary and alternative medicine: a primer. Fam Pract Manag 2001;8(3):37–42.

11. Buyukyilmaz F, Asti T. The effect of relaxation techniques and back massage on pain and anxiety in Turkish total hip or knee arthroplasty patients. Pain Manag Nurs 2013;14(3):143–54.

12. Topolska M, Chrzan S, Sapula R, et al. Evaluation of the effectiveness of therapeutic massage in patients with neck pain. Ortop Traumatol Rehabil 2012;14(2):115–24.

13. Lopez-Sendin N, Alburquerque-Sendin F, Cleland JA, et al. Effects of physical therapy on pain and mood in patients with terminal cancer: a pilot randomized clinical trial. J Altern Complement Med 2012;18(5):480–6.

14. An LX, Chen X, Ren XJ, et al. Electro-acupuncture decreases postoperative pain and improves recovery in patients undergoing a supratentorial craniotomy. Am J Chin Med 2014;42(5):1099–109.

15. Chen CC, Yang CC, Hu CC, et al. Acupuncture for pain relief after total knee arthroplasty: a randomized controlled trial. Reg Anesth Pain Med 2014;40:31–6.

16. Sun Y, Gan TJ, Dubose JW, et al. Acupuncture and related techniques for postoperative pain: a systematic review of randomized controlled trials. Br J Anaesth 2008;101(2):151–60.

17. Hinman RS, McCrory P, Pirotta M, et al. Acupuncture for chronic knee pain: a randomized clinical trial. JAMA 2014;312(13):1313–22.

18. Manheimer E, Cheng K, Linde K, et al. Acupuncture for peripheral joint osteoarthritis. Cochrane Database Syst Rev 2010;(1):CD001977.

19. Ezzo J, Berman B, Hadhazy VA, et al. Is acupuncture effective for the treatment of chronic pain? A systematic review. Pain 2000;86(3):217–25.

20. Vickers AJ, Cronin AM, Maschino AC, et al. Acupuncture for chronic pain: individual patient data meta-analysis. Arch Intern Med 2012;172(19):1444–53.

21. Yang B, Yi G, Hong W, et al. Efficacy of acupuncture on fibromyalgia syndrome: a meta-analysis. J Tradit Chin Med 2014;34(4):381–91.

22. Shin HK, Jeong SJ, Lee MS, et al. Adverse events attributed to traditional Korean medical practices: 1999-2010. Bull World Health Organ 2013;91(8):569–75.

23. Sahbaie P, Sun Y, Liang DY, et al. Curcumin treatment attenuates pain and enhances functional recovery after incision. Anesth Analg 2014;118(6):1336–44.

24. Di Pierro F, Settembre R. Safety and efficacy of an add-on therapy with curcumin phytosome and piperine and/or lipoic acid in subjects with a diagnosis of peripheral neuropathy treated with dexibuprofen. J Pain Res 2013;6:497–503.

25. Panahi Y, Rahimnia AR, Sharafi M, et al. Curcuminoid treatment for knee osteoarthritis: a randomized double-blind placebo-controlled trial. Phytother Res 2014;28:1625–31.

26. Kuptniratsaikul V, Dajpratham P, Taechaarpornkul W, et al. Efficacy and safety of Curcuma domestica extracts compared with ibuprofen in patients with knee osteoarthritis: a multicenter study. Clin Interv Aging 2014;9:451–8.

27. Chandrasekaran CV, Sundarajan K, Edwin JR, et al. Immune-stimulatory and anti-inflammatory activities of Curcuma longa extract and its polysaccharide fraction. Pharmacognosy Res 2013;5(2):71–9.

28. Kim DC, Kim SH, Choi BH, et al. Curcuma longa extract protects against gastric ulcers by blocking H2 histamine receptors. Biol Pharm Bull 2005;28(12):2220–4.

29. Thamlikitkul V, Bunyapraphatsara N, Dechatiwongse T, et al. Randomized double blind study of curcuma domestica Val. for dyspepsia. J Med Assoc Thai 1989;72(11):613–20.

30. Thong-Ngam D, Choochuai S, Patumraj S, et al. Curcumin prevents indomethacin-induced gastropathy in rats. World J Gastroenterol 2012;18(13): 1479–84.

31. Thomson M, Al-Qattan KK, Al-Sawan SM, et al. The use of ginger (Zingiber officinale Rosc.) as a potential anti-inflammatory and antithrombotic agent. Prostaglandins Leukot Essent Fatty Acids 2002;67(6):475–8.

32. Terry R, Posadzki P, Watson LK, et al. The use of ginger (Zingiber officinale) for the treatment of pain: a systematic review of clinical trials. Pain Med 2011; 12(12):1808–18.

33. Altman RD, Marcussen KC. Effects of a ginger extract on knee pain in patients with osteoarthritis. Arthritis Rheum 2001;44(11):2531–8.

34. Bartels EM, Folmer VN, Bliddal H, et al. Efficacy and safety of ginger in osteoarthritis patients: a meta-analysis of randomized placebo-controlled trials. Osteoarthritis Cartilage 2014;23:13–21.

35. Wigler I, Grotto I, Caspi D, et al. The effects of Zintona EC (a ginger extract) on symptomatic gonarthritis. Osteoarthritis Cartilage 2003;11(11):783–9.

36. Chopra A, Lavin P, Patwardhan B, et al. 32-week randomized, placebo-controlled clinical evaluation of RA-11, an Ayurvedic drug, on osteoarthritis of the knees. J Clin Rheumatol 2004;10(5):236–45.

37. Nieman DC, Shanely RA, Luo B, et al. A commercialized dietary supplement alleviates joint pain in community adults: a double-blind, placebo-controlled community trial. Nutr J 2013;12(1):154.

38. Chopra A, Saluja M, Tillu G, et al. Comparable efficacy of standardized Ayurveda formulation and hydroxychloroquine sulfate (HCQS) in the treatment of rheumatoid arthritis (RA): a randomized investigator-blind controlled study. Clin Rheumatol 2012;31(2):259–69.

39. Mandal P, Das A, Majumdar S, et al. The efficacy of ginger added to ondansetron for preventing postoperative nausea and vomiting in ambulatory surgery. Pharmacognosy Res 2014;6(1):52–7.

40. Dabaghzadeh F, Khalili H, Dashti-Khavidaki S, et al. Ginger for prevention of antiretroviral-induced nausea and vomiting: a randomized clinical trial. Expert Opin Drug Saf 2014;13(7):859–66.

41. Matthews A, Haas DM, O'Mathuna DP, et al. Interventions for nausea and vomiting in early pregnancy. Cochrane Database Syst Rev 2014;(3):CD007575.

42. Viljoen E, Visser J, Koen N, et al. A systematic review and meta-analysis of the effect and safety of ginger in the treatment of pregnancy-associated nausea and vomiting. Nutr J 2014;13:20.

43. Marx WM, Teleni L, McCarthy AL, et al. Ginger (Zingiber officinale) and chemotherapy-induced nausea and vomiting: a systematic literature review. Nutr Rev 2013;71(4):245–54.

44. Ryan JL, Heckler CE, Roscoe JA, et al. Ginger (Zingiber officinale) reduces acute chemotherapy-induced nausea: a URCC CCOP study of 576 patients. Support Care Cancer 2012;20(7):1479–89.

45. Marx W, McCarthy AL, Ried K, et al. Can ginger ameliorate chemotherapy-induced nausea? Protocol of a randomized double blind, placebo-controlled trial. BMC Complement Altern Med 2014;14:134.

46. Garcia MK, McQuade J, Haddad R, et al. Systematic review of acupuncture in cancer care: a synthesis of the evidence. J Clin Oncol 2013;31(7):952–60.

47. Shen Y, Liu L, Chiang JS, et al. Randomized, placebo-controlled trial of K1 acupoint acustimulation to prevent cisplatin-induced or oxaliplatin-induced nausea. Cancer 2014;121:84–92.

48. Dundee JW, Yang J. Prolongation of the antiemetic action of P6 acupuncture by acupressure in patients having cancer chemotherapy. J R Soc Med 1990;83(6):360–2.

49. Molassiotis A, Helin AM, Dabbour R, et al. The effects of P6 acupressure in the prophylaxis of chemotherapy-related nausea and vomiting in breast cancer patients. Complement Ther Med 2007;15(1):3–12.

50. Taspinar A, Sirin A. Effect of acupressure on chemotherapy-induced nausea and vomiting in gynecologic cancer patients in Turkey. Eur J Oncol Nurs 2010;14(1):49–54.

51. Allais G, Rolando S, Castagnoli Gabellari I, et al. Acupressure in the control of migraine-associated nausea. Neurol Sci 2012;33(Suppl 1):S207–10.

52. Nilsson I, Karlsson A, Lindgren L, et al. The efficacy of P6 acupressure with seaband in reducing postoperative nausea and vomiting in patients undergoing craniotomy: a randomized, double-blinded, placebo-controlled study. J Neurosurg Anesthesiol 2014;27:42–50.

53. Windle PE, Borromeo A, Robles H, et al. The effects of acupressure on the incidence of postoperative nausea and vomiting in postsurgical patients. J Perianesth Nurs 2001;16(3):158–62.

54. Manusirivithaya S, Sripramote M, Tangjitgamol S, et al. Antiemetic effect of ginger in gynecologic oncology patients receiving cisplatin. Int J Gynecol Cancer 2004;14(6):1063–9.

55. Hornyak M, Voderholzer U, Hohagen F, et al. Magnesium therapy for periodic leg movements-related insomnia and restless legs syndrome: an open pilot study. Sleep 1998;21(5):501–5.

56. Lakhan SE, Vieira KF. Nutritional and herbal supplements for anxiety and anxiety-related disorders: systematic review. Nutr J 2010;9:42.

57. Rondanelli M, Opizzi A, Monteferrario F, et al. The effect of melatonin, magnesium, and zinc on primary insomnia in long-term care facility residents in Italy: a double-blind, placebo-controlled clinical trial. J Am Geriatr Soc 2011;59(1):82–90.

58. Pandi-Perumal SR, Srinivasan V, Spence DW, et al. Role of the melatonin system in the control of sleep: therapeutic implications. CNS Drugs 2007;21(12):995–1018.

59. Abbasi B, Kimiagar M, Sadeghniiat K, et al. The effect of magnesium supplementation on primary insomnia in elderly: a double-blind placebo-controlled clinical trial. J Res Med Sci 2012;17(12):1161–9.

60. Orphan Drug Designations and Approvals. 2014. Available at: http://www.accessdata.fda.gov/scripts/opdlisting/oopd/index.cfm. Accessed December 01, 2014.

61. Buscemi N, Vandermeer B, Hooton N, et al. The efficacy and safety of exogenous melatonin for primary sleep disorders. A meta-analysis. J Gen Intern Med 2005;20(12):1151–8.

62. Garfinkel D, Laudon M, Nof D, et al. Improvement of sleep quality in elderly people by controlled-release melatonin. Lancet 1995;346(8974):541–4.

63. Haimov I, Lavie P, Laudon M, et al. Melatonin replacement therapy of elderly insomniacs. Sleep 1995;18(7):598–603.

64. Obayashi K, Saeki K, Tone N, et al. Lower melatonin secretion in older females: gender differences independent of light exposure profiles. J Epidemiol 2015; 25(1):38–43.

65. Bent S, Padula A, Moore D, et al. Valerian for sleep: a systematic review and meta-analysis. Am J Med 2006;119(12):1005–12.

66. Hellum BH, Nilsen OG. The in vitro inhibitory potential of trade herbal products on human CYP2D6-mediated metabolism and the influence of ethanol. Basic Clin Pharmacol Toxicol 2007;101(5):350–8.

67. Gurley BJ, Gardner SF, Hubbard MA, et al. In vivo effects of goldenseal, kava kava, black cohosh, and valerian on human cytochrome P450 1A2, 2D6, 2E1, and 3A4/5 phenotypes. Clin Pharmacol Ther 2005;77(5):415–26.

68. Cheuk DK, Yeung WF, Chung KF, et al. Acupuncture for insomnia. Cochrane Database Syst Rev 2012;(9):CD005472.

69. Gao X, Xu C, Wang P, et al. Curative effect of acupuncture and moxibustion on insomnia: a randomized clinical trial. J Tradit Chin Med 2013;33(4):428–32.

70. Tu JH, Chung WC, Yang CY, et al. A comparison between acupuncture versus zolpidem in the treatment of primary insomnia. Asian J Psychiatr 2012;5(3): 231–5.

71. Zhao K. Acupuncture for the treatment of insomnia. Int Rev Neurobiol 2013;111: 217–34.

72. Barton DL, Liu H, Dakhil SR, et al. Wisconsin Ginseng (Panax quinquefolius) to improve cancer-related fatigue: a randomized, double-blind trial, N07C2. J Natl Cancer Inst 2013;105(16):1230–8.

73. Finnegan-John J, Molassiotis A, Richardson A, et al. A systematic review of complementary and alternative medicine interventions for the management of cancer-related fatigue. Integr Cancer Ther 2013;12(4):276–90.

74. Lo LC, Chen CY, Chen ST, et al. Therapeutic efficacy of traditional Chinese medicine, Shen-Mai San, in cancer patients undergoing chemotherapy or radiotherapy: study protocol for a randomized, double-blind, placebo-controlled trial. Trials 2012;13:232.

75. Barton DL, Soori GS, Bauer BA, et al. Pilot study of Panax quinquefolius (American ginseng) to improve cancer-related fatigue: a randomized, double-blind, dose-finding evaluation: NCCTG trial N03CA. Support Care Cancer 2010; 18(2):179–87.

76. Mao JJ, Farrar JT, Bruner D, et al. Electroacupuncture for fatigue, sleep, and psychological distress in breast cancer patients with aromatase inhibitor-related arthralgia: a randomized trial. Cancer 2014;120:3744–51.

77. Towler P, Molassiotis A, Brearley SG. What is the evidence for the use of acupuncture as an intervention for symptom management in cancer supportive and palliative care: an integrative overview of reviews. Support Care Cancer 2013;21(10):2913–23.

78. Deng G, Chan Y, Sjoberg D, et al. Acupuncture for the treatment of post-chemotherapy chronic fatigue: a randomized, blinded, sham-controlled trial. Support Care Cancer 2013;21(6):1735–41.

79. Bader S, Weber M, Becker G. Is the pharmacological treatment of constipation in palliative care evidence based?: a systematic literature review. Schmerz 2012;26(5):568–86 [in German].

80. Ishihara M, Ikesue H, Matsunaga H, et al. A multi-institutional study analyzing effect of prophylactic medication for prevention of opioid-induced gastrointestinal dysfunction. Clin J Pain 2012;28(5):373–81.

81. Munshi R, Bhalerao S, Rathi P, et al. An open-label, prospective clinical study to evaluate the efficacy and safety of TLPL/AY/01/2008 in the management of functional constipation. J Ayurveda Integr Med 2011;2(3):144–52.

82. Fleming V, Wade WE. A review of laxative therapies for treatment of chronic constipation in older adults. Am J Geriatr Pharmacother 2010;8(6):514–50.

83. Miles CL, Fellowes D, Goodman ML, et al. Laxatives for the management of constipation in palliative care patients. Cochrane Database Syst Rev 2006;(4):CD003448.

84. Mitchell JM, Mengs U, McPherson S, et al. An oral carcinogenicity and toxicity study of senna (Tinnevelly senna fruits) in the rat. Arch Toxicol 2006;80(1):34–44.

85. Morales MA, Hernandez D, Bustamante S, et al. Is senna laxative use associated to cathartic colon, genotoxicity, or carcinogenicity? J Toxicol 2009;2009:287247.

86. Keefer L, Taft TH, Kiebles JL, et al. Gut-directed hypnotherapy significantly augments clinical remission in quiescent ulcerative colitis. Aliment Pharmacol Ther 2013;38(7):761–71.

87. Moser G, Tragner S, Gajowniczek EE, et al. Long-term success of GUT-directed group hypnosis for patients with refractory irritable bowel syndrome: a randomized controlled trial. Am J Gastroenterol 2013;108(4):602–9.

88. Dimidi E, Christodoulides S, Fragkos KC, et al. The effect of probiotics on functional constipation in adults: a systematic review and meta-analysis of randomized controlled trials. Am J Clin Nutr 2014;100(4):1075–84.

89. Malaguarnera G, Leggio F, Vacante M, et al. Probiotics in the gastrointestinal diseases of the elderly. J Nutr Health Aging 2012;16(4):402–10.

90. Redman MG, Ward EJ, Phillips RS. The efficacy and safety of probiotics in people with cancer: a systematic review. Ann Oncol 2014;25(10):1919–29.

91. Santino I, Alari A, Bono S, et al. Saccharomyces cerevisiae fungemia, a possible consequence of the treatment of Clostridium difficile colitis with a probioticum. Int J Immunopathol Pharmacol 2014;27(1):143–6.

92. Van den Nieuwboer M, Brummer RJ, Guarner F, et al. The administration of probiotics and synbiotics in immune compromised adults: is it safe? Benef Microbes 2015;6:3–17.

93. Emery EA, Ahmad S, Koethe JD, et al. Banana flakes control diarrhea in enterally fed patients. Nutr Clin Pract 1997;12(2):72–5.

94. Natural standard: the authority on integrative medicine. 2014. Available at: https://naturalmedicines.therapeuticresearch.com. Accessed December 01, 2014.

95. Natural medicines comprehensive database. 2014. Available at: http://naturaldatabase.therapeuticresearch.com. Accessed December 01, 2014.

96. Warde P, Kroll B, O'Sullivan B, et al. A phase II study of Biotene in the treatment of postradiation xerostomia in patients with head and neck cancer. Support Care Cancer 2000;8(3):203–8.

97. Roozbeh J, Hashempur MH, Heydari M. Use of herbal remedies among patients undergoing hemodialysis. Iran J Kidney Dis 2013;7(6):492–5.

98. Vegh A, Lanko E, Fittler A, et al. Identification and evaluation of drug-supplement interactions in Hungarian hospital patients. Int J Clin Pharm 2014; 36(2):451–9.
99. Navarro VJ, Barnhart H, Bonkovsky HL, et al. Liver injury from herbals and dietary supplements in the U.S. Drug-induced Liver Injury Network. Hepatology 2014;60(4):1399–408.
100. NSF international: the public health and safety organization. 2014. Available at: http://www.nsf.org. Accessed December 01, 2014.
101. U.S. Pharmacopeial Convention. 2014. Available at: http://www.usp.org. Accessed December 01, 2014.

Palliative Care in the Ambulatory Geriatric Practice

Thomas E. Finucane, MD*, Olivia Nirmalasari, MD,
Antonio Graham, DO

KEYWORDS

• Advance care planning • Pain management • Geriatrics • Elderly

KEY POINTS

- Clinicians should recognize the "the widespread and deeply held desire not to be dead (WDHDNTBD)", inquire about understanding of illness, and approach advance care planning with great care.
- For chronic pain, clinicians should reject the idea of a pain-free drug-centered cure; nonpharmacologic approaches should be emphasized.
- The risks of chronic narcotics and their common failure in eliminating pain and improving function should be explicitly stated.

INTRODUCTION

"Geriatrics" and "palliative care" are each poorly defined and the 2 overlap greatly. In both, early diagnosis and aggressive treatment of disease have become less important. In both, the patient's family and community may be more essential to the patient's care. In both, patient goals and careful attention to symptoms are central (although patient centeredness and symptom management are part of good care for nearly all patients). In both, the difficult task of suggesting explicitly to patients that they are mortal must often be undertaken.

Geriatrics care is mindful of the progressive frailty, vulnerability, comorbidity, and cognitive impairment that often accompany advancing age, with the correspondingly increased risks from medical treatments. Palliative care focuses on quality of life and symptom management, especially in patients with serious illness or limited life expectancy.

Division of Gerontology and Geriatric Medicine, Johns Hopkins University School of Medicine, Beacham Ambulatory Care Clinic, Johns Hopkins Bayview Medical Center, 5505 Hopkins Bayview Circle, John R. Burton Pavilion, Baltimore, MD 21224, USA
* Corresponding author.
E-mail address: tfinucan@jhmi.edu

Clin Geriatr Med 31 (2015) 193–206
http://dx.doi.org/10.1016/j.cger.2015.01.008
0749-0690/15/$ – see front matter © 2015 Elsevier Inc. All rights reserved.

In this article, we focus on 2 important topics: (1) advance planning and limitations of therapy in geriatrics and in palliative care and (2) pain management in the frail elderly.

In Part 1, we discuss the tempo of decision making. Palliative care consultants often see patients with acute or subacute life-threatening illness, whereas patients in ambulatory geriatrics tend to be more stable. The close relationship between palliative care and hospice means that patients may expect a discussion about limiting life-sustaining treatments. In ambulatory geriatrics, initiating such a discussion can be extremely fraught, and decision making often develops more gradually.

In Part 2, we suggest an approach to pain management in the frail elderly. For patients receiving palliative care, the long-term complications of narcotics may be limited and the need for narcotic pain relief clearer. In ambulatory geriatrics, chronic narcotics are clear and present dangers, and their effectiveness is uncertain.

We emphasize that commonalities shared by the 2 specialties are far greater than their distinctions. We emphasize too that our generalizations about vulnerable elders and patients with life-threatening illnesses are suspect in many ways. People can be unpredictable when confronted with the unimaginable. What is more, the 2 fields are changing rapidly. In 20 years, when Baby Boomers are the old-old, ambulatory geriatrics and palliative care will look very different. And it will be very difficult to know the reasons for the change.

PART 1: PLANNING ABOUT DYING: AMBULATORY GERIATRICS AND PALLIATIVE CARE

Two fundamental principles outline the paths to medical decision making for patients with life-threatening illness. The first is that life is the greatest good. If circumstances are uncertain, the default action should be to preserve life. The second and equally compelling principle is autonomy, in particular "Everyone has the right to say 'Keep your hands off me.'"[1] Tension may arise when patients who have capacity to make decisions are asked the "palliative care question": will you choose a focus on comfort and dignity with a greater chance of death or will you choose burdensome treatments that may help you live longer? A second, arguably more difficult set of problems arises when caring for patients who cannot make decisions.

Unwanted Conversations

Although death is thus far the universal fate of all humans, most of us retain a strange and powerful reluctance to imagine ourselves dead and to engage in explicit planning about medical events that will lead to that stage. In a qualitative, longitudinal study of 20 housebound, chronically ill, community-dwelling elders with an expected survival of less than 2 years, 13 had wills and 19 had funeral plans, but "Our patients were least likely to envision and help to plan for a period of chronic serious illness when death is not certain. It is precisely in this interval that the most difficult decisions often arise."[2] Two factors make it difficult for patients to plan for the contingencies of serious, potentially fatal illness. The first is technical; physicians cannot predict the future. In "Characterizing predictive models of mortality for older adults and their validation for use in clinical practice," Minne and colleagues[3] conclude "their use is premature." Of 193 models, only 4 were validated in more than 2 studies. Fox and colleagues,[4] using detailed data from SUPPORT on 2607 severely ill patients who had survived hospitalization, tried to identify those who would die in the next 6 months. In this large sample, many seriously ill patients "never experience a time during which they are clearly dying of their disease."

Parenthetically, this inability to provide good prognostic information for most patients leads to a necessarily incoherent use of the popular trope of "end-of-life care." A systematic review of "Evidence for improving palliative care at the end of life" both "chronic, eventually fatal illness with ambiguous prognosis (eg, advanced dementia)" and "clinician assessment of 'active dying' or 'patient readiness,'" were included as definition of "end of life," "but no precise definitions or performance characteristics of these terms have been published."[5]

Frank discussions about management during life-threatening illness are further complicated by "the widespread and deeply held desire not to be dead (WDHDNTBD)."[6] Patients who previously expressed disdain for aggressive treatment near death commonly seek aggressive treatment once death comes into view. This is especially well-documented in patients with advanced cancer.[7]   .

Being teased about the possibility of being one century old, a 96-year-old man pointed out that "The only people who REALLY want to live to be 100 … are all in their late 90's."

A Mexican saying has it that *los toros se ven major desde la barrera* (roughly, "bulls look a lot better from behind the barrier").

Confronting the desire not to be dead is uncomfortable for physicians and patients; nearly three-quarters of patients on chemotherapy for metastatic colon and lung cancer "did not report understanding that chemotherapy was not at all likely to cure their cancer."[8] The rate of misunderstanding was greatest among those who rated their physician most favorably. The authors conclude, "Physicians may be able to improve patients' understanding, but this may come at the cost of patients' satisfaction with them."[8] The name of the widely used POLST is a clear attempt to sidestep the issue. Physician Orders for Life-Sustaining Treatment were developed to document physician orders against life-sustaining therapy. According to Kübler-Ross, "death is still a fearful, frightening happening, and the fear of death is a universal fear even if we think we have mastered it on several levels."[9]

The Conversation's Context

One major difference between ambulatory geriatrics and palliative care is the relationship in which discussions to limit care occurs. The geriatrician–patient relationship is focused on an implicit agreement to minimize risks and improve health. In a continuity clinic visit, discussions about limiting treatment might seem incongruous and threatening, especially for patients with a recent worsening of medical status. In contrast, palliative care consultants meet patients explicitly, in many cases, to fashion an "exit strategy." The name "palliative care" in itself signals that limitations on prognosis and treatment may be part of the conversation. Asking a patient with cancer to consider discontinuing statin therapy might be straightforward in the latter conversation and highly menacing in the former.

After a "code status" discussion, a cognitively intact 84-year-old woman who was doing well during a hospitalization for pneumonia chose to have a do not resuscitate (DNR) order entered into her chart. The geriatrician provided reassurance that this was largely a formality and that he did not expect the order to be relevant for years to come. The patient replied, "Well, I didn't either. Otherwise I wouldn't have given you that answer."

This difference may lead some clinicians and commentators working in palliative care to portray advance care planning as straightforward and perhaps obligatory. Similarly, patients entering hospice have reconciled themselves, at least to some extent, to less aggressive treatment and a foreseeable death. These reconciled patients are more likely to agree to enter hospice and the higher satisfaction seen among patients and their families who are cared for in hospice in part owing to this selection bias. (The great work done by hospice staff is of course a wonderful thing to behold.)

Capacity?

Any in-depth discussion of capacity is beyond the scope of this article. We offer 2 brief suggestions. First, determination of decisional capacity usually depends on what decisions are needed. A person may have capacity to play chess but not tennis, and to order dinner but not decide about the risk of leaving the hospital. Second, as noted by Roth and associates,[10] "The search for a single test of competence is a search for the Holy Grail. Unless it is realized that there is no magical definition of competency to make decisions about treatment, the search for an acceptable test will never end ... judgments (about competence) reflect social considerations and societal biases as much as the reflect matters of law and medicine."

For patients who are conversational, decisional capacity can best be determined during a conversation about the decision. If the patient makes a consistent decision without coercion and it is among the set of choices that the physician considers reasonable, in most cases there is little further evaluation. In cases where there is contention or unclarity, asking the patient to discuss the consequences of her choice and the consequences of the competing alternatives often provides insight as to whether the choice is meaningful. In many cases, however, the definition of "reasonable" is subject to "social considerations and societal biases."

Advance Directives: Context

Because of the variable and uncertain tempo of death's approach and the widespread and deeply held desire not to be dead (WDHDNTBD), determination of capacity to make decisions to forgo life-sustaining treatment is especially fraught. For patients who can be clearly determined to lack decisional capacity, different questions arise; decisions that might lead to the patient's death will be made by someone other than the patient. Dispute resolution in this arena does not depend generally on finding the right answer. What we seek is a fair and transparent way to decide among the morally acceptable possibilities.

The tragic case of Robert Wendland is important. Mr. Wendland had repeatedly told his family that he would not want to be kept alive unless he were able to provide for his family, take care of himself, and enjoy life. He then survived a terrible traumatic brain injury at age 42 and recovered only to the point of severe cognitive loss and complete physical dependency. "At his highest level of function between February and July, 1995, Robert was able to do such things as throw and catch a ball, operate an electric wheelchair with assistance, turn pages, draw circles, draw an 'R' and perform 2-step command... [h]e was able to respond appropriately to the command 'close your eyes and open them when I say the number 3'. He could choose a requested color block out of four color blocks. He could set the right peg in a pegboard. Augmented communication was met with inconsistent success. He remained unable to vocalize. Eye blinking was successfully used as a communication mode for a while, however no consistent method of communication was developed."[11]

When his feeding tube became dislodged 2 years after the injury, his wife refused permission to replace it. His mother felt that he should be fed. Long court proceedings ensued. At one point the court sent a physician to Mr. Wendland. The dialogue shown in **Box 1** was documented.[11] Two people with strong personal commitment to him reached opposite conclusions about what was right.

Box 1
Dialogue between physician and Robert Wendland

After a series of questions about Robert's physical state, such as "Are you sitting up?" and "Are you lying down?" that Robert seemed to answer correctly "most times," Dr Kass asked the following questions and received the following answers:

"Do you have pain?" "Yes."

"Do your legs hurt?" "No."

"Does your buttocks hurt?" "No."

"Do you want us to leave you alone?" "Yes."

"Do you want more therapy?" "No."

"Do you want to get into the chair?" "Yes."

"Do you want to go back to bed?" "No."

"Do you want to die?" No answer.

"Are you angry" "Yes."

"At somebody?" "No."

From Cal. 4th Supreme Court of California Cases. Conservatorship of Wendland. 2001. Available at: http://law.justia.com/cases/california/supreme-court/4th/26/519.html. Accessed February 12, 2015.

Planning About an Unimaginable Future

Mr. Wendland's history demonstrates the instability of some advance directives. Although he had in advance left clear guidance to forgo treatment, he may have changed his mind when he faced the precise situation. Perhaps for this reason, every state limits contingency-based advance directives, often called Living Wills. In Maryland, for example, Living Wills can only be used to limit life-sustaining treatment if 1 of 3 qualifying conditions is present: terminal condition, persistent vegetative state, and severe, progressive dementia causing complete physical dependency. The limitations vary by state, but no state permits glib statements by healthy people to be binding years later; a qualifying condition must be present. For this reason, the legal authority of the POLST and the "Five Wishes" documents may vary by jurisdiction.

Many states provide a second method for leaving guidance in advance. Rather than identifying specific conditions as "worse than death" the person may designate a substitute decision maker and delegate authority to that person. These designated substitutes, with real-time information about patient-specific burdens and benefits, are given wide authority over decision making in most jurisdictions. An ideal health care agent would love and know the patient well and be available, strong, and dedicated to helping. In some, jurisdictions the agent, a designated substitute, has far broader authority than the default substitute or "next of kin," whereas in others the difference is less.

Nomenclature is also highly inconsistent. Some terms for the designated substitute include health care agent, surrogate, proxy, or "durable power of attorney for health care." (There is also great variability in how the default is named; proxy, surrogate, substitute and many other confusing, overlapping, and sometimes contradictory terminologies are in use.) Careful understanding of local language and law is important.

As Ambulatory Geriatrics Care Transitions Toward Palliative Care

Because of the difficult nature of the topic, discussions about goals of care with patients who have complex multimorbidity and frailty should often be considered a process in ambulatory geriatrics, whereas such discussions may be more decisive in palliative care context.[12]

For both specialties, family meetings are an essential tool in decision making, particularly during advanced disease. In preparation, a comfortable, private meeting place and setting are optimal. Timing should allow inclusion of companions important to the patient. The physician should know medical facts, the decisions to be made, and other goals of the meeting.[12] Adequate time should be allowed. The following are examples of themes that may help facilitate the discussion with patients and their families.

- What is your understanding of your illness?[13]
- Who are the most important people in your life?
- What are the most important things to you as your disease advances?
- Do you understand the options of treatment versus nontreatment?

Open-ended questions can allow patients greater latitude in expressing their understanding and goals. Perhaps even more important, the ability to sit in silence can be highly valuable. (Mozart may have said, "Notes are silver. Rests are gold.")

Information about options for community support—including medical assistant, sitter, and/or home health; Senior Day Care; local services; and the services of Medicare-certified Hospice—will be necessary for many decisions.[12,14]

Medicare Hospice eligibility depends on the physician's finding of a life expectancy of 6 months or less if the disease follows its usual course and on the patient's willingness to relinquish Medicare-reimbursed services that focus on cure or prolongation of life. A free mobile application such as Hospice in a Minute (https://itunes.apple.com/us/app/hopsice-in-a-minute/id511997344?mt=8) can be used as a guide to help clinicians determine hospice eligibility. Medicare Hospice benefits include physician and nurse services, which includes a home health aide for 4 hours per day on average for 3 days a week, respite care, social workers and physical and occupational therapies. Medications and durable medical equipment may be provided when appropriate, including a hospital bed and supplemental oxygen.[12,14] Quality of care varies among hospice providers.

Hospice also provides spiritual support regardless of faith and provides up to 12 months of spiritual support for family members.[14] Spiritual and emotional support from one's faith community can improve the quality of life for patients and families as death approaches.[12] Hospice services can also provide for bereaved families after the patient's death.

Although some people fear "hospice" and may see it as giving up on the patient and sentencing the patient to death, some studies show that survival of patients who use hospice is higher than those who do not, even after controlling for confounders.[15,16] Directly addressing this perspective, whether with patient, family, or both, is sometimes important in achieving best care for the patient. Hospice can provide care in multiple settings, that is, in nursing homes, as an inpatient, and in the home. Eligibility for inpatient care varies by hospice provider.

If a patient dies at home, family members may call one's practice and report the death. In most jurisdictions, a physician may sign the death certificate, and the family may call the funeral home to make arrangement, although practices are variable among jurisdictions. Family members may request an autopsy and this is handled differently in different locales as well. In the ambulatory geriatric setting, unexpected death can sometimes present difficult decisions.

Both geriatricians and palliative care specialists care for patients who are in the transition from a state of combat, battling, or at least resisting the disease, to a state of reconciliation and an acceptance that death is near and always inevitable. The primary distinction is the tempo of the transition and approach to death. The transitions are as individual and complex as the patients (and the people around them). Very few decisions are final.

PART 2: MANAGEMENT OF CHRONIC PAIN IN OUTPATIENT ELDERLY PATIENTS

Pain is experienced by each individual differently, modified by an individual's memories, expectations and emotions.[17] Using combined psychophysical assessment and functional MRI, Koyama and colleagues[18] demonstrated that manipulation of a subject's expectation of pain affected both the subjective experience of pain and the activation of pain-related brain regions. The individual's unique genotype, physical pathology, socioeconomic factors, and cognitive and behavioral factors may all affect the experience of pain.[19]

Prevalence and Characteristics of Pain

About two-thirds of elderly community-dwelling residents report experiencing some degree of pain within the past month, with about one-half of them reporting having daily pain.[20] Among terminally ill patients, the prevalence of pain varies from 36% to 75% in different studies.[21–24] Recent observational study suggests that the prevalence of pain during the last one year of life has increased, however the prevalence of moderate or severe pain did not change.[25] One study found "no association between the type of terminal disease and degree of pain" experienced,[24] disputing the common notion that nonmalignant disease is somehow less painful.

Analgesia: Use, Misuse, and Death

Pain management lies at the core of holistic patient care. The notion that pain is undertreated[26–29] has contributed to pressure on medical practitioners to prescribe more "painkillers." The medical use of opiates has increased at least 10-fold in the past 20 years.[30]

> "Americans, constituting only 4.6% of the world's population, consume 80% of the global opioid supply, and 99% of the global hydrocodone supply."[31]

Deaths from prescription opioid analgesics have risen steadily at rates faster than those from cocaine or heroin (**Fig. 1**), and they are now one of the leading causes of unintentional injury and/or death in United States.[30]

Death rates from opioid analgesic poisoning have increased each year by 18% from 1999 to 2006; however, the rate slowed down since 2006, with only a 3% increase.[32] Data from National Statistics also show that death from opioid analgesic poisoning often involves concomitant use of other drugs, most commonly benzodiazepines, which were present in about one-third of the opioid analgesic-related deaths in 2011 (**Fig. 2**).[32] Death from opiate overdose is most prevalent between ages 45 to 54, with a drastic decline after 54 years of age (**Fig. 3**).[32] The decline may be owing to age-related changes, differences in life-histories among the cohorts of patients (a "generation gap"), or other causes or combinations of causes. Future epidemiologic studies may confirm the cohort effect as an explanation, may show that overall use tends to fall in older age with each generation, or may show that prescription narcotic use has risen sharply owing to a secular trend such as pharmaceutical advertising. Recent epidemiologic data further highlight the increasing trend of prescription

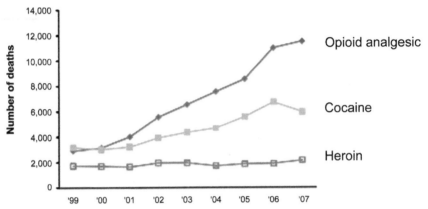

Fig. 1. Unintentional drug overdose deaths by major type of drug, United States, 1999 to 2007. (*From* Centers for Disease Control and Prevention. Unintentional drug poisoning in the United States CDC; 2010. Available at: http://www.cdc.gov/HomeandRecreationalSafety/pdf/poison-issue-brief.pdf. Accessed February 12, 2015.)

analgesic abuse among the elderly. Data from the Substance Abuse and Mental Health Administration (SAMHSA) suggest that 2.8 million seniors in United States abuse prescription drugs, and this number is expected to reach more than 4.4 million by 2020.[33]

Pain Management

> A woman in her 20s was brought to the emergency department by a coworker for acute abdominal pain. Responding to the emergency physician's questions, the patient reported intermittent right lower abdominal pain that lasted for 5 to 10 minutes per episode. Asked to rate the pain, the patient replied "9 to 10 out of 10." Shortly thereafter a nurse arrived with intravenous medication. The patient asked what the medicine was and was told that it was intravenous morphine to ease the pain so that the patient could lie still during the CT. The patient had never taken narcotics before. She politely asked to be given acetaminophen instead. The emergency room doctor complied but joked, "if someone were to see your chart, they might think that I'm being mean for giving you just acetaminophen for this degree of pain. This is a 'quality' issue."

The balance between the benefits and the harms of aggressive pain control may fall differently in ambulatory geriatrics than it does in palliative care. For patients with serious illness, severe pain, and a discretely limited life expectancy, best treatment is likely to include narcotics than for patients with no obvious physical cause and a relatively longer life expectancy. There is no "one size fits all" approach for pain control. The concept of individualized patient care in this situation cannot be overemphasized. Further, as the tempo of clinic visits and the ongoing campaign for more aggressive pain control accelerate, clinicians often fail to discuss alternative treatments and provide education about efficacy and potential harm before jumping to drug therapy.

Not all patients who are in pain want additional treatment.[24,34] One study found that "Although *half of terminally ill patients* experienced *moderate to severe pain, only 30%*

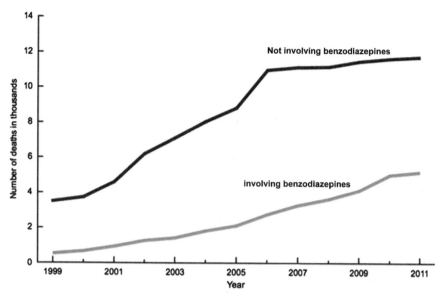

Fig. 2. Number of opioid-analgesic poisoning deaths, by involvement of benzodiazepines: United States, 1999 to 2011. (*From* Chen LH, Hedegaard H, Warner M. Drug-poisoning deaths involving opioid analgesics: United States, 1999–2011. NCHS Data Brief 2014;166:1–8. Available at: http://www.cdc.gov/nchs/data/databriefs/db166.pdf; CDC/NCHS, National Vital Statistics System, Mortality File.)

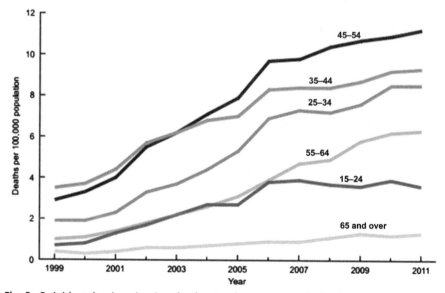

Fig. 3. Opioid-analgesic poisoning death rates, by age group: United States, 1999 to 2011. (*From* Chen LH, Hedegaard H, Warner M. Drug-poisoning deaths involving opioid analgesics: United States, 1999–2011. NCHS Data Brief 2014;166:1–8. Available at: http://www.cdc.gov/nchs/data/databriefs/db166.pdf; CDC/NCHS, National Vital Statistics System, Mortality File.)

of them wanted additional *pain treatment from their primary-care* physician."[24] Fear of addiction, exaggerated perceptions of the side effects of analgesics, and the burdens of polypharmacy are some reasons that patients fail to seek medical help for their pain.[24]

Routine screening for pain has not been shown to improve the quality of pain management,[35] but a careful assessment likely may. Initial pain assessments should include a detailed history of its characteristics, such as sites, onset period and level, history of injury, associated or contributing factors, previous medications, and impact on physiologic and functional status. The management of pain should include a meticulous and compassionate discussion about patient's goals and preferences, carefully weighing the risks and benefits of each regimen while matching his/her expectations with realistic goals. As a general rule, older patient have increased sensitivity to analgesics and thus may require lower doses. There should be frequent reassessment of pain control and careful titration of the regimen as necessary.

Management of Chronic Noncancer Pain

Chronic noncancer pain has been defined as pain that last longer than 3 months or beyond the expected period of tissue healing.[36] An extensive review of chronic noncancer pain, not limited to the elderly, suggested that "none of the most commonly prescribed treatment regimens are, by themselves, sufficient to eliminate pain and to have a major effect on physical and emotional function in most patients with chronic pain."[37] Although this reality is somber, optimal pain management for our patients remains a central goal. This extensive review further emphasized the need for individualized treatment and suggested that multimodality treatments may be required for better pain control. Herein we discuss commonly use pharmacologic and nonpharmacologic modalities for chronic noncancer pain management.

Pharmacologic Treatment

In many clinical situations, the clinician's dilemma is in choosing between narcotics and nonsteroidal anti-inflammatory drugs (NSAIDs). Both tend to be safe if used carefully in the short term. Both have very serious adverse effects if used chronically.

Opioids

An extensive review suggested that, compared with other analgesics, on average opioids result in similar reduction in pain but less improvement in overall function.[38] In addition, an elderly patient is more prone to develop confusion, cognitive impairment, and other adverse physical effects of opioids, making their long-term use problematic.

Nonsteroidal anti-inflammatory drugs

Oral NSAIDs are effective for the management of chronic inflammatory pain[39] and short-term relief for low back pain[40]; however, chronic use should be avoided owing to increased risk of gastrointestinal bleeding, peptic ulcer disease, and renal injury. Topical NSAIDs show potential benefit for chronic musculoskeletal pain with fewer systemic side effects; however, formulation can influence efficacy.[41]

Acetaminophen

Acetaminophen is recommended as the first-line therapy for less-than-severe pain. Liver toxicity remains a danger. Although uncommon,[42] concern for liver toxicity has led to increasingly stringent regulation by the US Food and Drug Administration. For frail patients and those with a history of alcohol use or hepatic insufficiency, maximum doses should be reduce to 3 g, or even 2 g in selected patients.

Antidepressant and antiseizure medications

Evidence is particularly strong for use in neuropathic pain[43,44] but neurologic side effects are commonly observed.

Muscle relaxants

No clear role has been shown for the agents in the treatment of chronic noncancer pain.

Topical agents

Topical agents have the potential advantage of fewer systemic side effects with potential benefit for short-term neuropathic and musculoskeletal pain.[41,45,46]

Interventional therapy

Interventional therapy, such as permanent intrathecal opioid therapy, is shown to provide at least short-term improvement in cancer pain reduction and functional level with less drug-related toxicity[47,48]; however, serious adverse events and high costs may limit its use. They are rarely used in our practice.

Nonpharmacologic Treatment

Physical therapy

There is evidence of benefit in patients with knee and shoulder pain,[49] but no good evidence available for patients with hip pain.[50]

Acupuncture

Acupuncture has possible benefits in chronic nonspecific musculoskeletal pain, osteoarthritis, chronic headache, or shoulder pain.[51]

Interdisciplinary pain rehabilitation program

An interdisciplinary pain rehabilitation program shows good evidence for pain reduction,[52] but resources for referral many be limited in many areas. Palliative care specialists and geriatricians share the same principles of pain management with goal of improving patient's quality of life by mitigating suffering. Complete pain relief is rare and the importance of function should be emphasized. An interdisciplinary approach is essential, as it always is in ambulatory geriatrics and in palliative care.

SUMMARY

Geriatrics and palliative care are poorly defined and often overlapping specialties. They both focus on end-of-life care and patients' goals and symptoms. They both require conversations about prognosis, advance directives, and death. These conversations are not one-time events but rather an interactive, dynamic process between patient and clinician. One should note that patients may change their mind about more aggressive treatment as death approaches; this is owing to "the widespread and deeply held desire not to be dead (WDHDNTBD)."[6]

In addition to end-of-life care, geriatrics and palliative care frequently involve pain management. In the frail elderly, pain management is complex, and there is no "one size fits all" strategy. For chronic noncancer pain, the long-term use of narcotics carries significant risk and often fails in eliminating pain or improving function. The idea of a pain-free drug-centered cure is more of myth than a reality and should be rejected. Geriatrics and palliative care can provide invaluable service to patients through careful discussion of patients' goals and symptoms, planning for death, and thoughtful pain management.

REFERENCES

1. Goldstein A. Court's decision on help with suicide leaves doctors in a gray zone. Available at: Washingtonpost.com. 1997; Friday, June 27. p. A18. Available at: http://www.washingtonpost.com/wp-srv/national/longterm/supcourt/stories/062797e.htm. Accessed February 12, 2015.
2. Carrese JA, Mullaney JL, Faden RR, et al. Planning for death but not serious future illness: qualitative study of housebound elderly patients. BMJ 2002; 325(7356):125.
3. Minne L, Ludikhuize J, de Rooij SE, et al. Characterizing predictive models of mortality for older adults and their validation for use in clinical practice. J Am Geriatr Soc 2011;59(6):1110–5.
4. Fox E, Landrum-McNiff K, Zhong Z, et al. Evaluation of prognostic criteria for determining hospice eligibility in patients with advanced lung, heart, or liver disease. Support investigators. Study to understand prognoses and preferences for outcomes and risks of treatments. JAMA 1999;282(17):1638–45.
5. Lorenz KA, Lynn J, Dy SM, et al. Evidence for improving palliative care at the end of life: a systematic review. Ann Intern Med 2008;148(2):147–59.
6. Finucane TE. How gravely ill becomes dying: a key to end-of-life care. JAMA 1999;282(17):1670–2.
7. Matsuyama R, Reddy S, Smith TJ. Why do patients choose chemotherapy near the end of life? A review of the perspective of those facing death from cancer. J Clin Oncol 2006;24(21):3490–6.
8. Weeks JC, Catalano PJ, Cronin A, et al. Patients' expectations about effects of chemotherapy for advanced cancer. N Engl J Med 2012;367(17):1616–25.
9. Kübler-Ross E. On death and dying. New York: Routledge; 1968. ISBN 0-415-04015-9.
10. Roth LH, Meisel A, Lidz CW. Tests of competency to consent to treatment. Am J Psychiatry 1977;134(3):279–84.
11. Available at: http://law.justia.com/cases/california/supreme-court/4th/26/519.html. Accessed February 12, 2015.
12. Morrison RS, Meier DE. Clinical practice. palliative care. N Engl J Med 2004; 350(25):2582–90.
13. Morris DA, Johnson KS, Ammarell N, et al. What is your understanding of your illness? A communication tool to explore patients' perspectives of living with advanced illness. J Gen Intern Med 2012;27(11):1460–6.
14. Report of the geriatrics-hospice and palliative medicine work group: American Geriatrics Society and American Academy of Hospice and Palliative Medicine Leadership Collaboration. J Am Geriatr Soc 2012;60(3):583–7.
15. Connor SR, Pyenson B, Fitch K, et al. Comparing hospice and nonhospice patient survival among patients who die within a three-year window. J Pain Symptom Manage 2007;33(3):238–46.
16. Saito AM, Landrum MB, Neville BA, et al. Hospice care and survival among elderly patients with lung cancer. J Palliat Med 2011;14(8):929–39.
17. Sternbach RA. Clinical aspects of pain. In: Sternbach RA, editor. The psychology of pain. New York: Raven Press; 1978. p. 223–39.
18. Koyama T, McHaffie JG, Laurienti PJ, et al. The subjective experience of pain: where expectations become reality. Proc Natl Acad Sci U S A 2005;102(36): 12950–5.
19. Gatchel RJ, Peng YB, Peters ML, et al. The biopsychosocial approach to chronic pain: scientific advances and future directions. Psychol Bull 2007;133(4):581–624.

20. Sawyer P, Bodner EV, Ritchie CS, et al. Pain and pain medication use in community-dwelling older adults. Am J Geriatr Pharmacother 2006;4(4):316–24.
21. Von Roenn JH, Cleeland CS, Gonin R, et al. Physician attitudes and practice in cancer pain management. A survey from the Eastern Cooperative Oncology Group. Ann Intern Med 1993;119(2):121–6.
22. Cleeland CS, Gonin R, Hatfield AK, et al. Pain and its treatment in outpatients with metastatic cancer. N Engl J Med 1994;330(9):592–6.
23. Bonica JJ. Cancer pain. In: Bonica JJ, editor. Pain. New York: Raven Press; 1980. p. 335–62.
24. Weiss SC, Emanuel LL, Fairclough DL, et al. Understanding the experience of pain in terminally ill patients. Lancet 2001;357(9265):1311–5.
25. Singer AE, Meeker D, Teno JM, et al. Symptom trends in the last year of life from 1998 to 2010: a cohort study. Annals of Internal Medicine 2015;162(3):175–83.
26. Scherder E, Oosterman J, Swaab D, et al. Recent developments in pain in dementia. BMJ 2005;330(7489):461–4.
27. Claxton RN, Blackhall L, Weisbord SD, et al. Undertreatment of symptoms in patients on maintenance hemodialysis. J Pain Symptom Manage 2010;39(2):211–8.
28. Deandrea S, Montanari M, Moja L, et al. Prevalence of undertreatment in cancer pain. a review of published literature. Ann Oncol 2008;19(12):1985–91.
29. Kim YE, Lee WW, Yun JY, et al. Musculoskeletal problems in Parkinson's disease: neglected issues. Parkinsonism Relat Disord 2013;19(7):666–9.
30. Unintentional drug poisoning in the United States. Centers for Disease Control and Prevention. 2010. Available at: http://www.cdc.gov/HomeandRecretionalSafety/pdf/poison-issue-brief.pdf. Accessed February 12, 2015.
31. Available at: http://www.asipp.org/documents/TESTIMONY-FROMEXECUTIVE COMMITTEE-RESPONDINGTOTHEPRESCRIPTIONDRUGEPIDEMIC-STRATEGIES FORREDUCI.pdf. Accessed February 12, 2015.
32. Chen LH, Hedegaard H, Warner M. Drug-poisoning deaths involving opioid analgesics: United States, 1999–2011. NCHS Data Brief 2014;166:1–8. Available at: http://www.cdc.gov/nchs/data/databriefs/db166.pdf.
33. Lowry F. Prescription opioid abuse in the elderly an urgent concern. Medscape Medical News from the 23rd Annual Meeting & Symposium of the American Academy of Addiction Psychiatry (AAAP). Aventura (FL), December 13, 2012.
34. Weeks JC, Cook EF, O'Day SJ, et al. Relationship between cancer patients' predictions of prognosis and their treatment preferences. JAMA 1998;279(21):1709–14.
35. Mularski RA, White-Chu F, Overbay D, et al. Measuring pain as the 5th vital sign does not improve quality of pain management. J Gen Intern Med 2006;21(6):607–12.
36. Turk DC, Okufuji A. Pain terms and taxonomies of pain. In: Fishman SM, Ballantyne JC, Rathmell JP, editors. Bonica's management of pain. 4th edition. New York: Lippincott Williams & Wilkins; 2009. p. 13–23.
37. Turk DC, Wilson HD, Cahana A. Treatment of chronic non-cancer pain. Lancet 2011;377(9784):2226–35.
38. Furlan AD, Sandoval JA, Mailis-Gagnon A, et al. Opioids for chronic noncancer pain: a meta-analysis of effectiveness and side effects. CMAJ 2006;174(11):1589–94.
39. Wienecke T, Gotzsche PC. Paracetamol versus nonsteroidal anti-inflammatory drugs for rheumatoid arthritis. Cochrane Database Syst Rev 2004;(1):CD003789.

40. Roelofs PD, Deyo RA, Koes BW, et al. Nonsteroidal anti-inflammatory drugs for low back pain: an updated Cochrane Review. Spine (Phila Pa 1976) 2008; 33(16):1766–74.
41. Derry S, Moore RA, Rabbie R. Topical NSAIDs for chronic musculoskeletal pain in adults. Cochrane Database Syst Rev 2012;(9):CD007400.
42. Bernal W, Wendon J. Acute liver failure. N Engl J Med 2013;369(26):2525–34.
43. Attal N, Cruccu G, Haanpaa M, et al. EFNS guidelines on pharmacological treatment of neuropathic pain. Eur J Neurol 2006;13(11):1153–69.
44. Dworkin RH, O'Connor AB, Audette J, et al. Recommendations for the pharmacological management of neuropathic pain: an overview and literature update. Mayo Clin Proc 2010;85(3 Suppl):S3–14.
45. Mason L, Moore RA, Edwards JE, et al. Systematic review of efficacy of topical rubefacients containing salicylates for the treatment of acute and chronic pain. BMJ 2004;328(7446):995.
46. Zacher J, Altman R, Bellamy N, et al. Topical diclofenac and its role in pain and inflammation: an evidence-based review. Curr Med Res Opin 2008;24(4):925–50.
47. Turner JA, Sears JM, Loeser JD. Programmable intrathecal opioid delivery systems for chronic noncancer pain: a systematic review of effectiveness and complications. Clin J Pain 2007;23(2):180–95.
48. Smith TJ, Coyne PJ, Staats PS, et al. An implantable drug delivery system (IDDS) for refractory cancer pain provides sustained pain control, less drug-related toxicity, and possibly better survival compared with comprehensive medical management (CMM). Ann Oncol 2005;16(5):825–33.
49. Juhl C, Christensen R, Roos EM, et al. Impact of exercise type and dose on pain and disability in knee osteoarthritis: a systematic review and meta-regression analysis of randomized controlled trials. Arthritis Rheumatol 2014;66(3):622–36.
50. Bennell KL, Egerton T, Martin J, et al. Effect of physical therapy on pain and function in patients with hip osteoarthritis: a randomized clinical trial. JAMA 2014; 311(19):1987–97.
51. Vickers AJ, Linde K. Acupuncture for chronic pain. JAMA 2014;311(9):955–6.
52. Morley S, Eccleston C, Williams A. Systematic review and meta-analysis of randomized controlled trials of cognitive behaviour therapy and behaviour therapy for chronic pain in adults, excluding headache. Pain 1999;80(1–2):1–13.

Interaction of Palliative Care and Primary Care

Amrita Ghosh, MD, PhD[a], Elizabeth Dzeng, MD, MPH, MPhil, MS[b,c], M. Jennifer Cheng, MD[a,*]

KEYWORDS

- Primary palliative care • Specialty palliative care • Referral

KEY POINTS

- Primary palliative care assessment includes a symptom assessment, assessing for moderate-to-severe distress, concerns regarding decision-making, and advance care planning.
- Advanced care planning and discussions about dying and palliative care in the outpatient setting by the PCP can improve end-of-life care outcomes.
- Shared decision-making has emerged as an ideal balance between respecting the patient's autonomy to make decisions, and the recognition of the clinician's medical expertise.
- Referral criteria algorithms are available for specialty palliative care referrals.

INTRODUCTION

Scope and Definition of Palliative Care

Palliative care is often believed to be synonymous with end-of-life care or required only after standard care interventions have failed to achieve a desired effect. In fact, earlier palliative care interventions have been shown to potentially increase quality of life, decrease cost of care, and improve survival of patients with metastatic cancer.[1] In 2001, standardization of palliative care with the goal of improving quality of care resulted in the formation of the National Consensus Project for Quality Palliative Care.

In 2009, the Accreditation Council for Graduate Medical Education recognized hospice and palliative medicine (HPM) as a subspecialty, and fellowship training for physicians is required to become HPM board eligible. Comparable certifications for nurses[2] and social workers[3,4] working in palliative care are also newly established

[a] Pain and Palliative Care Service, 10 Center Drive, Clinical Center, National Institutes of Health, Bethesda, MD 20892, USA; [b] Division of General Internal Medicine, Program in Palliative Care, The Johns Hopkins University School of Medicine, 600 North Wolfe Street, Blalock 359, Baltimore, MD 21287, USA; [c] University of Cambridge School of Clinical Medicine, Forvie Site, Robinson Way, Cambridge CB2 0SR, UK
* Corresponding author.
E-mail address: mok-chung.cheng@nih.gov

Clin Geriatr Med 31 (2015) 207–218
http://dx.doi.org/10.1016/j.cger.2015.01.001
0749-0690/15/$ – see front matter Published by Elsevier Inc.

geriatric.theclinics.com

or being developed. Accordingly, hospice programs and specialty palliative care programs have seen substantial growth[5,6] and increasingly, patients can receive palliative care services in outpatient settings, emergency and critical care departments, and acute care settings.[7]

The definition of palliative care by the Center to Advance Palliative Care (CAPC) is "focused on providing patients with relief from the symptoms, pain, and stress of a serious illness-whatever the diagnosis or prognosis. The goal is to improve quality of life for both the patient and the family." Furthermore, according to American Society of Clinical Oncology Provisional Clinical Opinion, palliative care is "focused on relief of suffering, in all of its dimensions."[1] Palliative care management focuses on symptom assessment and control while emphasizing honest and open communication with families and discussion of appropriate goals of care, especially in patients with advanced illness or significant symptom burden.

Why Primary Care Physicians Should Be Familiar with Palliative Care Approaches

Demand for palliative care specialists is growing rapidly and the number of providers may soon fall short of such demand. In 2008, a workforce task force was appointed by the American Academy of Hospice and Palliative Medicine to perform a needs assessment. The task force concluded that there were approximately 4400 HPM specialists available, whereas an estimated 4487 hospice and 10,810 palliative care physicians are required to staff current hospice and hospital-based palliative care programs. Current fellowship programs have the capacity to train approximately 180 HPM physicians annually. Taking into account the rate of retiring physicians, specialists in palliative care will most likely be unable to fill the annual need for replacement in even the lowest estimate-of-need scenario.[8]

Solutions to the deficiency of HPM physicians are needed to create a more sustainable model. One important strategy is to partner with primary care physicians (PCP) to address basic aspects of palliative care called primary palliative care.

Primary palliative care includes basic skills and competencies possessed by all physicians irrespective of specialty, whereas specialty palliative care includes secondary palliative care and tertiary palliative care. Secondary palliative care is provided by specialist consultants, whereas tertiary palliative care is provided at tertiary medical centers where specialists care for the most complex cases and where clinical care, research, and educational palliative care practices exist simultaneously. In contrast to primary palliative care, specialty palliative care includes managing complex or refractory symptoms and facilitating communication in challenging situations.[9]

Primary palliative care skills consist of elements that are at the heart of palliative care, including basic symptom management, aligning treatment plan with patient goals, and addressing patient suffering. By exercising primary palliative care skills, PCP strengthens existing therapeutic relationships, whereas referring to specialist palliative care services for all basic symptom management and psychosocial support may further fragment care.

Objectives for Primary Palliative Care in the Primary Care Setting

PCP are often the first medical provider patients seek out and are therefore in an excellent position to identify patients who are in need of primary or specialty palliative care services. Many PCP have worked with patients and families for many years and have the added benefit of well-established relationships. PCP are thus well positioned to identify patients that may benefit from early palliative strategies and to provide such care concurrently with life-prolonging interventions. Primary palliative care evaluation can include performing a symptom assessment, assessing for moderate-to-severe distress, addressing concerns regarding decision-making, and assisting with advance care planning.[10] Symptom assessment includes reviewing the more common symptoms and their impact on daily life as shown in **Table 1**. Important decision-making steps can be explored and should be triggered by changes in the disease state: when disease worsens, prognosis changes, after recent hospitalizations, or performance status declines. Useful questions include whether patients have a living will or advanced directive, explaining the benefits and risks of cardiopulmonary resuscitation, and identifying a medical decision-maker who would act on behalf of the patient's wishes.

PRIMARY PALLIATIVE CARE SKILL SET
Symptom-Based Management

PCPs are often the first called on to manage patients' basic symptoms. Therefore, completing a symptom assessment and learning the basic principles of symptom management are essential tools in a physician's tool box.

For example, chronic pain is a symptom that results in significant suffering and economic cost[11–13] and has been increasingly seen as a top national health priority.[14] After maximizing nonopioid pain medications, treatment of chronic severe pain may include the use of opioid medications. Another common symptom is depression. Depression in the outpatient setting is common and has impact on the patient's and family's suffering and quality of life. For outpatients, one or two screening questions can have greater than 80% sensitivity.[15–17] The sole screening question, "Are you depressed?" has been shown in cancer survivors to have a high negative predictive value, so screening for depression need not be an arduous time-consuming evaluation.[15,16]

Other disease- or treatment-related symptoms include nausea, fatigue, intestinal obstruction, and pain from bony lesions. Metoclopramide, haloperidol, or olanzapine can be used for cancer-related nausea[18]; American ginseng can improve fatigue[19]; and referral for radiation therapy for patients with pain from uncomplicated nonvertebral bone metastases is advisable.[20] Please refer to the article on symptom management in the older adult elsewhere in this issue for more in-depth discussions.

Performing a Spiritual Assessment

A spiritual assessment is a key part of primary palliative care, and involving spiritual care specialists, such as chaplains, for patients facing multiple comorbid conditions and high emotional burden can improve patient satisfaction.[21] When medical teams

Table 1
Common symptoms to review on symptom assessment

Symptoms	Assess Impact on Daily Life
Pain Tiredness Nausea Depression Anxiety Drowsiness Anorexia Constipation Dyspnea Secretions	1. On a scale from 1 to 10, 10 being the most severe [symptom], how would you rate your [symptom] right now? At its best? At its worse? What is a tolerable level for you? 2. How much impact does the [symptom] have on your daily life? 3. How bothersome is the [symptom]?

address spiritual care, patients with terminal illness are five times more likely to use hospice and have better quality-of-life scores.[22] A simple assessment tool is the Faith, Importance, Community, Address tool (**Box 1**),[23] or simply ask "Is religion or spirituality important to you?" Community connections to chaplains are essential when referrals are necessary.

Discussions Regarding Advanced Care Planning

Many of the challenges surrounding discussions of advanced care planning in the primary care setting revolve around practitioners' discomfort regarding discussions of death. Concerns revolve around broaching a subject that would cause distress, depression, or destroy hope.[24,25] A recent British study showed that 35% of general practitioners had not initiated a discussion of end-of-life wishes and that 79% agreed that the British public was uncomfortable discussing dying and death.[26] Most Americans want to die at home without pain or suffering, but most die in the hospital undergoing aggressive care.[27,28]

Advanced care planning and discussions about dying and palliative care in the outpatient setting by the PCP can improve end-of-life care outcomes. It is particularly important to convey prognosis accurately, because studies have shown that patients already tend to have an optimism bias toward the curative efficacy of palliative treatments.[29,30] Physicians similarly have been found to be overly optimistic in their prognostication.[31] Given these inherent societal and clinical challenges to discussing prognosis and death, greater comfort and skills regarding these difficult conversations can help counter these inherent biases.

Failure to accurately prognosticate can lead to poorer patient outcomes, such as underuse of hospice care, or underuse and overuse of appropriate preventative screening. Poor prognostication leads to delays in advanced care planning and conversations surrounding death. Many physicians do not feel comfortable prognosticating and studies have shown that physician prognostic accuracy can be poor.[32] One study showed that only 20% of predictions were accurate, overestimating survival by a factor of 5.3.[31] The discomfort physicians feel about prognostication is evident in conversations because prognosis is rarely discussed during these conversations.[33] Despite this, one study showed that 87% of surrogates still wanted physicians to discuss prognosis even if uncertain. Surrogates prefer this primarily because they understand that prognostic uncertainty is unavoidable, and that physicians' are

---

Box 1
Example questions for the Faith, Importance, Community, Address spiritual assessment tool

Faith	• "Do you come from a particular faith or spiritual background?"
	• "What things give you a sense of meaning in your life?"
Importance	• "Is your faith or spirituality important to you?"
	• "Do your beliefs play a role in your health?"
Community	• "Are you part of a faith or spiritual community?"
	• "Is there a group of people who are very important to you?"
Address	• "How can we help address your spiritual needs?"

Data from Borneman T, Ferrell B, Puchalski CM. Evaluation of the FICA tool for spiritual assessment. J Pain Symptom Manage 2010;40(2):163–73; with permission.

their only source of this important information, which is important for preparation of the bereavement process.[32]

Prognostic indices have been developed to help predict overall mortality in various patient groups, although there are limitations to many of them.[34] One such index is ePrognosis (eprognosis.ucsf.edu), which has been validated for use in predicting post-hospital mortality in older adults.[35] This index makes predictions based on such factors as functional status, comorbidities, and laboratory measures, such as creatinine.

Shared decision making has emerged as an ideal balance between respecting the patient's autonomy to make decisions, and the recognition of the clinician's medical expertise, which the patient should be given the opportunity to benefit from. Conversations surrounding advanced planning and palliative care should balance the patient's goals and values with the physician's understanding of the clinical situation and prognosis.

In American medicine today, many physicians are hesitant to provide recommendations because of concerns of infringing on a patient's autonomy. This fails to recognize that often patients want and require recommendations to make an informed decision.[33] Indeed, the American Medical Association and other leading ethical organizations state that providing professional recommendations is a necessary element to autonomous decision making.[36,37] Studies have shown that patients and surrogates vary in the degree of support they want to make regarding end-of-life decisions. One study showed that 56% of surrogates preferred to receive a recommendation and 42% preferred not to.[38] This variation highlights the need to ask patients early on in the conversation how they prefer to receive their information, how much information they desire, and whether they would like to hear the physician's recommendation.

An important first step is to establish an appropriate private setting and environment for these conversations. If possible, ensure that there is sufficient time for the conversation while minimizing potential interruptions. Ask if family members or others should be present, and ensure that all are comfortable. Conversations should subsequently begin with an elicitation of the patient's understanding of their illness and prognosis, and clarification of accurate clinical information where necessary. Subsequent discussion should focus on the patient's expectations, goals, and values. If you perceive the patient's expectations and hopes to be overly optimistic, this is a good time to clarify and manage expectations. At this time, the physician can state their recommendation for the best course of action, and together with the patient, establish a consensus on the best plan.[39]

In general, the physician should listen carefully, remain empathetic, and be responsive to emotions to establish the trust necessary for a productive, respectful conversation.[25,40] Questions should be open-ended and nonjudgmental. In one study comparing expert internists in communications or bioethics with the average physician, experts spent twice as much time listening and were less verbally dominant. The expert physicians gave less information but spent more time building partnerships and asking psychosocial and lifestyle questions.[41]

Resuscitation status and the initiation of a do-not-resuscitate order is an important element of this goals of care conversation, although physicians must also be careful to recognize that resuscitation is but one component of a series of important decisions that must be made.[42] Such forms as the Medical Order for Life Sustaining Therapies and Physician Order for Life Sustaining Therapies recognize the need to expand the focus of end-of-life conversations beyond resuscitation.[43] Furthermore, it is important to recognize that although advanced care planning is important, it is an imperfect tool that must be readdressed and recrafted through time. A patient's preferences can change depending on the circumstance so it is important that these advanced planning decisions are reviewed frequently and are responsive to change.[40]

Continuing Relationships with Patients After Referral

If patients do ultimately require specialty palliative care referral, maintaining and emphasizing the primacy of the relationship between PCP and patient is important for continuity of patient care. Regular communication between teams is essential to providing care consistent with patient goals and wishes, to coordination of care, and to avoid redundancy.[44,45]

When to Refer to Specialty Palliative Care Services

Referral criteria algorithms are increasingly being used as a means of identifying patients in need of referral for specialty services.[46] Variables, such as disease state, severe symptoms, and psychosocial emotional impact of illness, are included in decision algorithms.[1,47]

Referral in the Inpatient Setting

The consultation service is the most common form of palliative care service delivery in acute care hospitals. Difficult-to-manage symptoms, complex family dynamics, and challenging care decisions regarding the use of life-sustaining therapies are all reasons to consider specialty palliative care.[48–51] In 2008 to 2010, CAPC compiled a list of suggested triggers for in-patient palliative care consultation services.[52–54] Key principles from the consensus statement stress the following: specialty-level palliative care professionals should be used in complex cases, every hospital should develop a systematic approach to ensure that patients who require but have unmet palliative care needs are identified and supported in a timely fashion, patients should undergo a screening for palliative care assessment as part of day-to-day care, and hospitals should have a specialty-level palliative care service available. **Fig. 1** summarizes

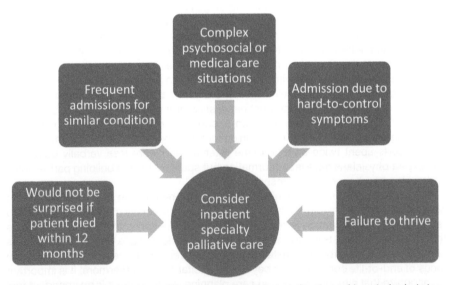

Fig. 1. Criteria for considering palliative care assessment at the time of hospital admission. (*Data from* Weissman DE, Meier DE. Identifying patients in need of a palliative care assessment in the hospital setting: a consensus report from the Center to Advance Palliative Care. J Palliat Med 2011;14(1):17–23.)

triggers from the CAPC Consensus Report for medical providers to consider consulting specialty palliative care at the time of hospital admission.[46]

Referral in the Outpatient Setting

A wide variety of models for palliative care exist for patients seeking palliative care services in the outpatient setting. However, outpatient palliative care programs are relatively infrequent, small,[55] affiliated with cancer centers, and have varied availability from half-day per week to 5 full days weekly.[56] Studies regarding which outpatient palliative care model is best remain ambiguous but clinical practice guidelines do exist.[57] Much of the same criteria for inpatient referrals can be extrapolated to palliative care consultation in the outpatient setting. In inpatient and outpatient settings, palliative care is ideally provided by an interdisciplinary team, which may include physicians, mid-level providers, social workers, nurses, spiritual care, rehabilitation medicine, nutrition, and other health professionals.[58] In fact, inclusion of social workers greatly facilitated completion of advance directives in one study.[59]

Three models exist for outpatient palliative care services. The first is a consultation model: recommendations are conveyed to the primary team but the palliative care team does not prescribe medications. The second is an embedded or integrated palliative care model. This is a collaborative model where the palliative care team takes the lead in managing symptoms while other physicians manage disease-modifying therapy.[60] In this model, communication between teams is essential to provide consistent management plans to the patient and avoid mixed messages. The third and final model is one where the palliative care team takes over all aspects of care including diagnosis, management, and prescriptions for all health issues, including the disease that triggered a palliative care referral. Care in this model is not common but may be the favored strategy for patients who decline curative antineoplastic treatment or may not be eligible for such therapies. Patients may or may not be simultaneously enrolled in hospice services and care may be provided in many settings including the home, nursing home, or care facility.[59]

Outpatient palliative care consultation visits may be lengthy, ranging from 60 to 120 minutes.[56,61,62] The content of an outpatient palliative care visit depends on the reasons for referral, the patient, and the palliative care providers. In addition to the standard history and physical, the typical palliative care assessment includes the domains shown in **Box 2**.[44]

When to Consider Hospice Referral

When patients have 3 to 6 months to live, an informational hospice referral should be made.[1] Indicators of 6-month mortality in advanced noncancer illnesses vary by disease and can facilitate the practitioner in initiating goals of care discussions with the patient.[63]

Patients with nonmalignant conditions but with high burden of disease may be a challenge in estimating life expectancy. Prognostic uncertainty and lack of evidence concerning efficacy of treatments in far advanced disease may add to general practitioners' uncertainty regarding patients requiring palliative treatment strategies. A screening question for identifying patients who may benefit from palliative strategies includes asking, "Would I be surprised if my patient were to die in the next 12 months?"[64] Tools exist to predict survival of less than or equal to 6 months for patients with and without cancer.[63,65] Decline in performance status, weight loss or anorexia, and any malignant effusion should all trigger consideration for hospice.

Box 2
Domains of palliative care assessment

Physical symptoms	• Pain, nausea, fatigue, cough, constipation, dyspnea, insomnia, depression, anxiety, issues with intimacy, and so forth
Psychosocial	• Preferred way of coping, cultural issues, education/employment, impact of illness, significant relationships, sources of stress and support
Assistance with practical needs	• Living situation, caregiver needs, financial issues, access to health care, transportation, nutrition
Spiritual care	• Faith, importance of spirituality, connection to faith community, need to address spirituality in context of medical care
Support for decision making	• Discuss and facilitate advance care planning, goals of and preferences for care
• End-of-life care

Data from Von Roenn JH, Temel J. The integration of palliative care and oncology: the evidence. Oncology (Williston Park) 2011;25(13):1258–60, 62, 64–5.

To receive Medicare hospice benefit, a PCP and the hospice medical director must certify that the patient has an expected prognosis of 6 months or less, based on documented criteria that vary depending on illness. In general, there should be progression of disease as evidenced by symptoms, test results, or imaging. The Medicare hospice benefit provides end-of-life care to terminally ill patients and their families and hospice eligibility guidelines were extended to those dying of noncancer diagnoses, including geriatric diseases, such as advanced dementia, and cardiovascular disease. Adult failure to thrive was a Medicare-supported hospice diagnosis until October 1, 2014.[66] A high-quality hospice program is usually Medicare certified, with staff trained in HPM; offers medical, nursing, social work, bereavement, and spiritual services; and engages in patient- and family-centered care.[67]

For many within the medical field, hospice is synonymous with specialty palliative care services. The primary goals of both groups are similar: to maximize quality of life, provide pain and symptom management, and provide psychosocial and spiritual support via an interdisciplinary team approach for patients and their families. The PCP often continues to provide overall medical care for hospice and palliative care patients while a hospice medical director and palliative care specialist provides expertise in disease-related symptom management.

Hospice services and specialty palliative care differs in that palliative care services may be delivered concurrently with curative or life-prolonging therapies, whereas with hospice enrollment, patients are choosing hospice care instead of other Medicare-covered benefits to treat their terminal illness.[67] This distinction, however, is evolving. The passage of the Patient Protection and Affordable Care Act of 2010 added new provisions allowing children access to hospice and curative care under the Children's Health Insurance Program[68] and establishing a 3-year Medicare hospice concurrent care demonstration program.

Ultimately, referrals to hospice must be in line with a patient's goals of care. When all available options are presented and not just the next step in medical management, discussions lead naturally to patient- and family-centered goals and quality of life. Drawing connections between patients' goals and services provided by hospice makes these conversations easier.[69]

SUMMARY

With ever-increasing demand for HPM physicians, primary care providers serve an integral role in providing primary palliative care. Primary palliative care skills, such as completing basic symptom and spiritual assessments and managing common symptoms, are essential in caring for the geriatric population, as is having competency in basic advanced care planning discussions. Specialty palliative care provides an extra layer of support for patients and PCP in managing refractory symptoms and navigating complex goals of care discussions. Knowing when to refer patients to palliative care and hospice services is important in maximizing their quality of life and providing aggressive symptom management throughout the entire disease course. The relationship between primary care and specialty palliative care will undoubtedly continue to grow and evolve and will continue to benefit patients and their caregivers.

REFERENCES

1. Smith TJ, Temin S, Alesi ER, et al. American Society of Clinical Oncology provisional clinical opinion: the integration of palliative care into standard oncology care. J Clin Oncol 2012;30(8):880–7.
2. National Board for Certification of Hospice and Palliative Nursing. History of palliative nursing. 2012. Available at: http://hpcc.advancingexpertcare.org/. Accessed February 11, 2015.
3. National Association of Social Workers. Advanced certified hospice and palliative social worker (ACHP-SW) credential applicant materials. 2012. Available at: http://preview.socialworkers.org/credentials/applications/achp-sw.pdf. Accessed February 11, 2015.
4. National Association of Social Workers. Certified hospice and palliative social worker (CHP-SW) credential applicant materials. 2012. Available at: http://preview.socialworkers.org/credentials/applications/chf-sw.pdf. Accessed February 11, 2015.
5. National Hospice and Palliative Care Organization. NHPCO facts and figures: hospice care in America. Available at: http://www.nhpco.org/files/public/Statistics_Research/2012_Facts_Figures.pdf. Accessed February 11, 2015.
6. Center to Advance Palliative Care. Analysis of US hospital palliative care programs, 2012 snapshot. Available at: http://www.capc.org/capc-growth-analysis-snapshot-2011.pdf. Accessed February 11, 2015.
7. Center to Advance Palliative Care. A state-by-state report care on access to palliative care in our nation's hospitals. 2010. Available at: http://www.capc.org/reportcard/. Accessed February 11, 2015.
8. Lupu D, American Academy of Hospice and Palliative Medicine Workforce Task Force. Estimate of current hospice and palliative medicine physician workforce shortage. J Pain Symptom Manage 2010;40(6):899–911.
9. Quill TE, Abernethy AP. Generalist plus specialist palliative care: creating a more sustainable model. N Engl J Med 2013;368(13):1173–5.
10. NCCN guidelines for supportive care. Available at: http://www.nccn.org/professionals/physician_gls/f_guidelines.asp#survivorship. Accessed February 11, 2015.
11. Gaskin DJ, Richard P. The economic costs of pain in the United States. J Pain 2012;13(8):715–24.
12. Gureje O, Von Korff M, Simon GE, et al. Persistent pain and well-being: a World Health Organization study in primary care. JAMA 1998;280(2):147–51.

13. Jackman RP, Purvis JM, Mallett BS. Chronic nonmalignant pain in primary care. Am Fam Physician 2008;78(10):1155–62.

14. Committee on Advancing Pain Research, Care, and Education; 2011. Institute of Medicine (US). Available at: http://www.iom.edu/Activities/PublicHealth/PainResearch.aspx. Accessed February 11, 2015.

15. Kroenke K, Spitzer RL, Williams JB. The Patient Health Questionnaire-2: validity of a two-item depression screener. Med Care 2003;41(11):1284–92.

16. Whooley MA, Avins AL, Miranda J, et al. Case-finding instruments for depression. two questions are as good as many. J Gen Intern Med 1997;12(7):439–45.

17. Lowe B, Kroenke K, Grafe K. Detecting and monitoring depression with a two-item questionnaire (PHQ-2). J Psychosom Res 2005;58(2):163–71.

18. Gupta M, Davis M, LeGrand S, et al. Nausea and vomiting in advanced cancer: the Cleveland Clinic protocol. J Support Oncol 2013;11(1):8–13.

19. Barton DL, Soori GS, Bauer BA, et al. Pilot study of panax quinquefolius (American ginseng) to improve cancer-related fatigue: a randomized, double-blind, dose-finding evaluation: NCCTG trial N03CA. Support Care Cancer 2010;18(2):179–87.

20. Expert Panel on Radiation Oncology-Bone Metastases, Lo SS, Lutz ST, et al. ACR appropriateness criteria (R) spinal bone metastases. J Palliat Med 2013;16(1):9–19.

21. Williams JA, Meltzer D, Arora V, et al. Attention to inpatients' religious and spiritual concerns: predictors and association with patient satisfaction. J Gen Intern Med 2011;26(11):1265–71.

22. Balboni TA, Balboni M, Enzinger AC, et al. Provision of spiritual support to patients with advanced cancer by religious communities and associations with medical care at the end of life. JAMA Intern Med 2013;173(12):1109–17.

23. Borneman T, Ferrell B, Puchalski CM. Evaluation of the FICA tool for spiritual assessment. J Pain Symptom Manage 2010;40(2):163–73.

24. Mack JW, Smith TJ. Reasons why physicians do not have discussions about poor prognosis, why it matters, and what can be improved. J Clin Oncol 2012;30(22):2715–7.

25. Von Roenn JH, von Gunten CF. Setting goals to maintain hope. J Clin Oncol 2003;21(3):570–4.

26. Wise J. Dying remains a taboo subject for patients and GPs, finds survey. BMJ 2012;344:e3356.

27. Institute of Medicine. Dying in America improving quality and honoring individual preferences near the end of life. 2014. Available at: www.iom.edu/Reports/2014/Dying-In-America-Improving-Quality-and-Honoring-Individual-Preferences-Near-the-End-of-Life.aspx. Accessed February 11, 2015.

28. Steinhauser KE, Christakis NA, Clipp EC, et al. Factors considered important at the end of life by patients, family, physicians, and other care providers. JAMA 2000;284(19):2476–82.

29. Weeks JC, Catalano PJ, Cronin A, et al. Patients' expectations about effects of chemotherapy for advanced cancer. N Engl J Med 2012;367(17):1616–25.

30. Smith TJ, Longo DL. Talking with patients about dying. N Engl J Med 2013;368(5):481.

31. Christakis NA, Lamont EB. Extent and determinants of error in doctors' prognoses in terminally ill patients: prospective cohort study. BMJ 2000;320(7233):469–72.

32. Evans LR, Boyd EA, Malvar G, et al. Surrogate decision-makers' perspectives on discussing prognosis in the face of uncertainty. Am J Respir Crit Care Med 2009;179(1):48–53.

33. Anderson WG, Chase R, Pantilat SZ, et al. Code status discussions between attending hospitalist physicians and medical patients at hospital admission. J Gen Intern Med 2011;26(4):359–66.
34. Yourman LC, Lee SJ, Schonberg MA, et al. Prognostic indices for older adults: a systematic review. JAMA 2012;307(2):182–92.
35. Walter LC, Brand RJ, Counsell SR, et al. Development and validation of a prognostic index for 1-year mortality in older adults after hospitalization. JAMA 2001;285(23):2987–94.
36. Guidelines for the appropriate use of do-not-resuscitate orders. Council on Ethical and Judicial Affairs, American Medical Association. JAMA 1991;265(14):1868–71.
37. The President's commission for the study of ethical problems in medicine and biomedical and behavioural research: deciding to forego life sustaining treatment. 1983. Available at: https://bioethicsarchive.georgetown.edu/pcbe/reports/past_commissions/. Accessed February 11, 2015.
38. White DB, Evans LR, Bautista CA, et al. Are physicians' recommendations to limit life support beneficial or burdensome? bringing empirical data to the debate. Am J Respir Crit Care Med 2009;180(4):320–5.
39. End of Life/Palliative education resource center (EPERC). #23 discussing DNR orders. 2009. Available at: www.eperc.mcw.edu/EPERC/FastFactsIndex/ff_023.htm. Accessed February 11, 2015.
40. Tulsky JA. Beyond advance directives: importance of communication skills at the end of life. JAMA 2005;294(3):359–65.
41. Roter DL, Larson S, Fischer GS, et al. Experts practice what they preach: a descriptive study of best and normative practices in end-of-life discussions. Arch Intern Med 2000;160(22):3477–85.
42. Billings JA. Getting the DNR. J Palliat Med 2012;15(12):1288–90.
43. Meier DE, Beresford L. POLST offers next stage in honoring patient preferences. J Palliat Med 2009;12(4):291–5.
44. Von Roenn JH, Temel J. The integration of palliative care and oncology: the evidence. Oncology (Williston Park) 2011;25(13):1258–60, 1262, 1264–5.
45. Weissman DE, von Gunten CF. Palliative care consultations as American football: full contact, or just touch? J Palliat Med 2012;15(4):378–80.
46. Weissman DE, Meier DE. Identifying patients in need of a palliative care assessment in the hospital setting: a consensus report from the center to advance palliative care. J Palliat Med 2011;14(1):17–23.
47. Temel JS, Greer JA, Muzikansky A, et al. Early palliative care for patients with metastatic non-small-cell lung cancer. N Engl J Med 2010;363(8):733–42.
48. von Gunten CF. Secondary and tertiary palliative care in US hospitals. JAMA 2002;287(7):875–81.
49. Weissman DE. Consultation in palliative medicine. Arch Intern Med 1997;157(7):733–7.
50. Campbell ML. Palliative care consultation in the intensive care unit. Crit Care Med 2006;34(11 Suppl):S355–8.
51. Abrahm JL, Callahan J, Rossetti K, et al. The impact of a hospice consultation team on the care of veterans with advanced cancer. J Pain Symptom Manage 1996;12(1):23–31.
52. Weissman DE, Morrison RS, Meier DE. Center to advance palliative care palliative care clinical care and customer satisfaction metrics consensus recommendations. J Palliat Med 2010;13(2):179–84.
53. Weissman DE, Meier DE. Center to advance palliative care inpatient unit operational metrics: consensus recommendations. J Palliat Med 2009;12(1):21–5.

54. Davies B, Sehring SA, Partridge JC, et al. Barriers to palliative care for children: perceptions of pediatric health care providers. Pediatrics 2008;121(2):282–8.
55. Rabow MW, Smith AK, Braun JL, et al. Outpatient palliative care practices. Arch Intern Med 2010;170(7):654–5.
56. Meier DE, Beresford L. Outpatient clinics are a new frontier for palliative care. J Palliat Med 2008;11(6):823–8.
57. National Consensus Project for Quality Palliative Care. Clinical practice guidelines for quality palliative care 3rd edition. 2013. Available at: http://www. nationalconsensusproject.org/NCP_Clinical_Practice_Guidelines_3rd_Edition.pdf. Accessed February 11, 2015.
58. Dennis K, Librach SL, Chow E. Palliative care and oncology: integration leads to better care. Oncology (Williston Park) 2011;25(13):1271–5.
59. Bookbinder M, Glajchen M, McHugh M, et al. Nurse practitioner-based models of specialist palliative care at home: sustainability and evaluation of feasibility. J Pain Symptom Manage 2010;41:25–34.
60. Debono DJ. Integration of palliative medicine into routine oncological care: what does the evidence show us? J Oncol Pract 2011;7(6):350–4.
61. Jacobsen J, Jackson V, Dahlin C, et al. Components of early outpatient palliative care consultation in patients with metastatic nonsmall cell lung cancer. J Palliat Med 2011;14(4):459–64.
62. Riechelmann RP, Krzyzanowska MK, O'Carroll A, et al. Symptom and medication profiles among cancer patients attending a palliative care clinic. Support Care Cancer 2007;15(12):1407–12.
63. Salpeter SR, Luo EJ, Malter DS, et al. Systematic review of noncancer presentations with a median survival of 6 months or less. Am J Med 2012;125(5):512.e1–6.
64. Murray SA, Boyd K, Sheikh A, et al. Developing primary palliative care. BMJ 2004;329(7474):1056–7.
65. Salpeter SR, Malter DS, Luo EJ, et al. Systematic review of cancer presentations with a median survival of six months or less. J Palliat Med 2012;15(2):175–85.
66. National Association for Home Care and Hospice. Available at: http://www.nahc. org/mobile/NAHCReport/nr130805_1/. Accessed February 11, 2015.
67. Teno JM, Connor SR. Referring a patient and family to high-quality palliative care at the close of life: "we met a new personality... with this level of compassion and empathy". JAMA 2009;301(6):651–9.
68. Patient Protection and Affordable Care Act (PPACA), public law 111–148. 2010. Available at: http://www.gpo.gov/fdsys/pkg/PLAW-111publ148/pdf/PLAW-111publ148.pdf. Accessed February 11, 2015.
69. Casarett D, Crowley R, Stevenson C, et al. Making difficult decisions about hospice enrollment: what do patients and families want to know? J Am Geriatr Soc 2005;53(2):249–54.

Communication with Older, Seriously Ill Patients

Liesbeth M. van Vliet, PhD[a],*, Elizabeth Lindenberger, MD[b],
Julia C.M. van Weert, PhD[c]

KEYWORDS

- Communication • Palliative care • Empathy • Information • Decision making
- Tailoring • Geriatrics • Surrogates

KEY POINTS

- Communication serves 3 core functions: (1) empathic behavior, (2) information provision, and (3) enabling decision making.
- Communication with older people poses specific barriers, because age is associated with cognitive, physical, and social changes.
- Empathic communication, including assuring a continued relationship, is an important prerequisite for optimal outcomes.
- Older people's abilities for information processing decreases, stressing the importance of tailoring information, and empathy facilitates information processing.
- Eliciting patients' goals of care—with or without the help of surrogates—is important to come to effective decision making.
- Surrogates need assistance when making decisions for patients although they also have their own caregiver needs for support and information.

INTRODUCTION

Communication is an essential palliative care skill and core element of effective care for patients with serious and life-limiting illness.[1] Effective communication by health care providers results in multiple positive patient and family outcomes. These include improved patient satisfaction,[2,3] information recall,[4–6] caregiver well-being and bereavement outcomes,[7] and lower costs of care.[8]

Disclosure Statements: All authors have no disclosures to be made.
[a] Department of Palliative Care, Policy and Rehabilitation, Cicely Saunders Institute, King's College London, Bessemer Road, London SE5 9PJ, UK; [b] Brookdale Department of Geriatrics and Palliative Medicine, Icahn School of Medicine at Mount Sinai, 10th Floor, Annenberg Building One Gustave L. Levy Place, Box 1070, New York, NY 10029, USA; [c] Amsterdam School of Communication Research/ASCoR, University of Amsterdam, Nieuwe Achtergracht 166, Amsterdam 1018 WV, The Netherlands
* Corresponding author.
E-mail address: Liesbeth.van_vliet@kcl.ac.uk

Clin Geriatr Med 31 (2015) 219–230
http://dx.doi.org/10.1016/j.cger.2015.01.007
0749-0690/15/$ – see front matter © 2015 Elsevier Inc. All rights reserved.

Scholars have proposed a variety of theoretic goals that effective communication can serve (see de Haes and Bensing[9] for an overview). The commonalities of the functions of communication center around 3 themes: (i) Empathic behavior (eg, building a relationship and responding to emotions); (ii) Information provision (in addition to gathering); (iii) Enabling decision making (in addition to implementation of treatment plans).

Patients desire to be seen as individuals instead of a bundle of symptoms.[10] They value the provision of clear and timely information[11] and often express a preference for some control over or involvement in treatment decisions.[12]

Despite these proposed common goals of skilled communication, patients differ in their communication needs, with age often mentioned as influencing preferences[13–15] as well as posing specific barriers to effective communication.[16] Although older patients form a heterogeneous group,[17] several elements might contribute to these posed barriers. As described in **Box 1**, aging is associated with cognitive, physical, and social changes. These changes (in)directly affect the way older people process information and make decisions and stress the importance of identifying strategies to promote effective communication with this group.

This article describes key components of effective communication in caring for older people with serious illness. Specific skills that are effective in 3 core functions of communication are described: (1) empathic behavior, (2) information provision, and (3) enabling decision making. Specifically, the needs of older patients and their surrogates/family caregivers are focused on, and strategies for overcoming potential communication barriers unique to this patient group are discussed.

EMPATHIC BEHAVIOR

The use of empathy is critical for building trust and relationships and is especially important as the disease progresses.[22] Empathic communication is associated with greater patient satisfaction,[2] decreased feelings of anxiety,[23] and better information recall.[5,6]

Patients frequently place high value on relationship with their clinicians and may fear being left alone when active treatment options are exhausted.[24] When clinicians stress their continued support and availability, this can profoundly influence patients' perceptions of communication.[25] Of course, such promises should be lived up to.

Although empathic communication, including reassurance about a continued relationship, is a critical component of patient care, the specific skills needed may be challenging for providers. The NURSE acronym[26–28] offers a scaffolding to promote empathic verbal communication during difficult conversations (described in **Table 1**

Box 1
Older people's unique characteristics contributing to communication barriers

- First, older people face functional declines,[18,19] such as hearing and vision loss, posing significant barriers to effective verbal and nonverbal communication
- Next, cognitive decline often occurs,[18,19] which can affect processing and recall of information[20,21]
- Of particular importance are situations of severe cognitive decline, such as in dementia, making elderly patients dependent on surrogates and family caregivers (often the same persons)
- Multimorbidity may lead to increasingly complex medical and also communicative situations[18]
- Lastly, social problems and isolation threaten older peoples' social network[19]

Table 1
Examples of providing empathic communication

Communication Style	Example
NURSE	
N—Name the emotion	"I can see you are really sad about this."
U—Understand	"I understand how tough it is for you to hear this."
R—Respect	"I admire how you have been dealing with this disease and all setbacks."
S—Support	"But whatever happens, we will be here for you. We will never leave you alone."
E—Explore emotion	"Tell me more about what you meant when you said you are scared."
Nonverbal communication	The use of eye contact[10] Sitting instead of standing when sharing bad news[29]

along with nonverbal communication examples contributing to the emitting of empathy).

When focusing specifically on older people, the level of unfulfilled psychological needs is often high[14] and older cancer patients experience more unfulfilled needs in affective communication than younger patients.[30] For example, they report a lack of performance in domains as "providing space for feelings and emotions" or "showing empathy."[31]

For older people, empathic communication and a good doctor-patient relationship may also facilitate information processing. According to the socioemotional selectivity theory, older adults use emotion-related goals to encode and memorize information, and information that gratifies emotional well-being seems better memorized.[32] In line with this theory, a trustful environment during patient-provider consultations is considered a prerequisite for reflection of older patients on the information provided and essential to enhance memory of information.[20] Encouraging responses to patients' emotional cues can positively influence older patients' recall of information.[4]

INFORMATION PROVISION

Furthermore, in addition to a need for empathy, patients need to be provided with information to understand their illness, to know what the future will bring, and to use for treatment decision making. Patients with serious illness need information about several topics, including their disease, treatment options, and life expectancy.[13] Many patients have difficulties processing and understanding provided information necessary to make informed decisions.[33]

Whether older patients desire less detailed information compared with younger people remains an unanswered question. Some studies suggest that a desire for detailed information regarding disease progression and prognosis may be less common among older people.[13] Other research has found only small differences between age groups in information and communication needs.[15] Whether or not they prefer less information, older patients tend to seek less information actively compared with younger ones and are often less proactive during consultations.[16] Consequently, they have much unmet information, communication, and support needs,[14] for instance, in discussing realistic expectations and receiving tailored communication.[31]

In addition, there is robust evidence that aging is associated with marked decline in effortful cognitive processes whereas implicit/automatic processes (eg, recognition memory) are relatively spared.[34] To illustrate, older adults in general, compared with younger adults, process information more slowly,[35] have a reduced working memory capacity,[36] and have more difficulty with controlling the regulation of cognition.[37] They also have more difficulty reproducing a large amount of information provided.[21]

Although these findings should not be interpreted as older people faring better by withholding information, they highlight the importance of assessing patients' information preferences and tailoring information to individual patients' needs and information processing abilities. Information may be tailored using several nonexhaustive approaches (outlined in **Table 2**). These suggestions can help with achieving patients receive information on the topics they prefer, and to the extent they prefer and can process.

Table 2 Approaches to tailor information	
Approach	**Explanation**
SPIKES	The SPIKES approach is a well-known and widely used model for discussing any bad news.[38] However, its acronym and suggestions are also appropriate for information discussion beyond bad news: • S stands for Setting up the encounter, including assessing who should be present at a conversation (eg, the patient, specific surrogates/family caregivers). • During the assessment of Perceptions, patients'/family caregivers' perceptions of the situation are assessed to determine how much information is known. • The I in SPIKES stands for Invitation or Information and includes determining patients' information needs before providing any (bad) news. Helpful sentences are, "Some patients prefer to receive as much information as possible, while others do not need to know everything, and some are in between. What kind of person are you generally?" • Next, the delivery of Knowledge should be conducted in line with assessed preferences. • E stands for Empathy—responding empathically/exploring emotions with empathy (see the NURSE acronym in **Table 1**). • Within the final S (Strategizing/Summarizing), information is summarized and strategies for next steps are outlined.
Ask-Tell-Ask	The Ask-Tell-Ask approach[26] describes an interactive way of providing and tailoring information in a wide range of settings: • The first Ask stands for asking patients what kind of information they prefer and what their perceptions are, using questions like, "What would you like to discuss today?" and "Would you like me to tell you about the test results we got in?" • After a response of the patient, the required information can be delivered under the Tell heading, in an easy understandable jargon-free manner.[20] • The last Ask stands for checking whether this was the information patients indeed wanted to receive, whether they have any other questions, and whether they understand the provided information. One way to check this is by using sentences, such as, "Could you please tell me in your own words what I just told you? This will help me ensure that I provided you all the right information."
Chunks	Another helpful suggestion for tailoring information is to make use of small chunks of information instead of a long monolog[26] followed by checking whether patients understood the information.[20]

ENABLING DECISION MAKING

A last goal that communication serves includes enabling appropriate decision making. Most patients, including older ones, prefer to be involved in decision making.[39] More involved patients have an increased understanding of treatment options, confidence in decisions made, and satisfaction with care provided,[40] while experiencing less decisional conflict.[41] This involvement might result in improved treatment compliance and better quality of life.[42] Many patients, however, find it difficult to participate in the decision making process,[40,43] sometimes because they do not want to[44] or because physicians do not invite them to.[45]

Involving patients in their preferred level of decision making can be done by eliciting their goals of care. Patients' goals commonly change over time as illness progresses and patients adjust to disease. Examples of patient goals include life prolongation, relief of suffering, or setting of death.[46,47] Patients may express different goals simultaneously (eg, cure and relief of symptoms). **Table 3** outlines a 2-step approach to elicit goals of care.

Once goals of care are elicited, treatment recommendations can be provided that best match a patient's goals. Simultaneous goals may be supported by encouraging "hope for the best, prepare for the worst."[48] **Table 4** outlines appropriate steps for making treatment recommendations.

Older adults, compared with younger individuals, generally use simpler and less systematic decision strategies.[49] They may prefer fewer choice options,[50] make decisions faster,[49] focus on positive information,[32] and have greater difficulty understanding information about available options.[51] Moreover, the decision making process is complicated by poor representation of older people in clinical trials (even when an upper age limit is not specified, the actual accrual of patients $\geq$70 years is often not in conformity with incidence data, e.g[52]), especially those with comorbidities, polypharmacy, and physical and/or cognitive impairments.[53] This indicates there is limited knowledge on objective risks of treatment options, stressing the importance of eliciting patients' goals of care in the decision making process.

Communication with Older Patients Lacking Capacity

Given the increased prevalence of cognitive impairments, including dementia, with age, it is critical to assess decisional capacity when discussing treatment decisions. Decisional capacity is decision-specific and changes over time. For example, many patients with mild dementia have the capacity for medical decision making. Other patients may have capacity for less risky/complex decisions but lack capacity for more complex decisions.

Table 3 Two-step approach to elicit goals of care	
Approach	**Examples**
1. Exploring what gives life meaning	"Before we talk about next steps, I wonder if you can tell me more about your life. What are the things that most give your life meaning?" "What do you enjoy." "What is most important to you if your time is limited?"
2. Identifying concerns	"What concerns do you have about the future?" "What is the hardest part of this for you and your family?"

Table 4
Recommending a treatment plan based on patient's goals

Steps	Examples of Language to Use
Confirm a shared understanding of patient's goals.	"Thank you for sharing that with me. What I am hearing is that it is very important to you to be home and to have your pain well controlled. Does that sound right?"
Ask permission to give recommendation (similar to the "I" in SPIKES).	"I have some ideas about how we can help meet these goals. Is it okay if I suggest some next steps?"
Provide recommendations (similar to the "K" in SPIKES).	"In order to maximize your time at home, I recommend that we plan for you to go home with services from a hospice team, who can treat your pain and help support you and your family."
Confirm shared understanding of the plan and next steps; emphasize support (similar to the last "S" in SPIKES).	"We have talked about a lot of things today. What are your thoughts about these next steps? What else concerns you?" "I will continue to be your physician and work closely with the hospice team to support you through this." "Is it okay if I check in with you again tomorrow morning?"

Data from Pantilat SZ, Anderson WG, Gonzales MJ, et al. Hospital-based palliative medicine: a practical, evidence-based approach. New York: John Wiley & Sons; 2015.

Physicians frequently miss a diagnosis of incapacity.[54] It may be assessed clinically by any physician, not exclusively psychiatrists. When assessing capacity, physicians should use simple language, avoid jargon, and focus on a particular decision. To demonstrate capacity to make a medical decision, the patient must

1. Understand the relevant information regarding the proposed test/treatment
2. Appreciate his/her situation, including the medical condition and potential consequences of each potential decision
3. Use reasoning to make a decision
4. Communicate his/her choice[54]

Communication with Surrogates

If patients lack capacity, communication about prognosis, goals of care, and treatment decisions occurs with surrogates (often family members/friends). Surrogate decision making occurs in approximately half of older hospitalized patients and includes either sole surrogate decision making or joint patient and surrogate decision making.[55] Even if patients lack capacity for complex decision making, they may still be able to express important goals and values, assisting the surrogate in making decisions.

When communicating with surrogates, it should be emphasized that their role is to make decisions as the patient would have made them and based on the patient's previously expressed goals and values. This role can be extremely difficult for surrogates, because the desire to honor the patient's goals and values may conflict with emotions, such as fear of responsibility or guilt for the patient's death, desire to avoid family conflict, and hope for the patient to recover.[56] **Table 5** describes suggestions to assist surrogates in this role.

Table 5	
Suggestions to assist surrogates making decisions	
Suggestion	**Example**
Bring the patient's "voice" into the decision making process.	Helpful phrases include, "What gave her life meaning?" and "Can you tell me what your mother would say if she were sitting her in the room with us now?"
Identify underlying emotion and respond with empathy, including offering support for the surrogate's commitment to the patient.	For example, if a family member says, "I want you to do everything!" it is important to identify the emotional context and offer empathy. An appropriate response to explore the emotion would be, "I can't imagine how difficult this must be for you. Can you tell me more about what you mean by 'everything?'"[57]

Family Caregivers' Needs

Irrespective of acting as surrogates, caregivers have unique needs that require effective communication. Family caregivers' increased emotional vulnerability has been discussed by Andershed.[58] Caregivers place high importance on a trusted continued relationship[58] and value expressions of nonabandonment.[59] The communication and information needs of family members/caregivers are often unmet.[31]

Family caregivers have needs for information in the same domains as patients regarding diagnosis, treatment, and prognosis.[58] Caregivers' information needs might diverge from patients' needs, however, when a disease progresses, with caregivers preferring more information and patients less.[13] When death becomes imminent, caregivers also need information about the dying phase, including how to take care of their loved one.[13,60]

Lastly, as discussed previously, family caregivers often become surrogate decision makers when patients' cognitive abilities decline. To ensure that both patients' and family caregivers' needs are being met, use of family conferences, including assessing caregivers' own needs, can be recommended.[60] Evidence of their effectiveness is emerging, especially in ICUs.[59]

Suggestions on Meeting Patients' and Family Caregivers' Needs

Although the importance of an empathic and continued relationship, tailored information, and shared decision making for patients and caregivers is widely documented, barriers are often experienced in meeting these needs.[20,31] **Box 2** proposes suggestions to ensure patients' and caregivers' needs are met and that their outcomes are improved.

CONCLUSION

To conclude, this article aims to provide insight and suggestions for effective communication with older people who are seriously ill and their family caregivers, focusing on 3 core functions of communication: (i) Empathic behavior, (ii) Information provision and (iii) Enabling decision making.

Patients and their family caregivers have needs for emotional support and information. Empathic communication is critical and can be provided using NURSE statements and assuring a continued relationship. Increasing age is associated with a

---

Box 2
Suggestions to meet patients' and caregivers' communication needs

1. Although effective and empathic communication does not always need to be time consuming,[23,25] consultations and building a relationship fair better when sufficient time is provided. This is especially important for older people, who, due to cognitive and physical declines, may need more time to absorb information[35,61] compared with their younger counterparts. Therefore, the authors stress the importance of providing clinicians with enough time to communicate with older people and their family caregivers.

2. The use of one professional who is the first contact point for patients is another helpful suggestion. This professional can liaise with different clinicians to provide patients up-to-date information that is not conflicting (especially relevant in case of multimorbidities) and can ensure a continued relationship.

3. As discussed previously, more attention should be given to communication with family caregivers, who can have a double role of surrogate decision making while also having their own needs. Because of the increase of older people, this group will grow as well, stressing the importance of meeting their (unmet) needs.

4. Given the rapidly increasing aging population, the demand for palliative care will progressively outweigh its provision by palliative care experts. So, the last recommendation is to ensure that communication training is offered and ideally mandated for all staff working with older patients with serious illness. They should also include nurses[20] and residential and care home staff who have much contact with older patients and their social network.

---

decrease in proactive information gathering alongside decreased information processing abilities, stressing the importance of tailoring information using approaches such as SPIKES, Ask-tell-Ask, and providing chunks of information. Moreover, empathy facilitates information processing. For effective decision making, assessing patients' goals of care is essential, where patients' can participate to different degrees, depending on capacity. In older age, surrogate decision making becomes increasingly important and surrogates need assistance in this difficult role while also having their own caregiver needs for support and information. Lastly, several suggestions to ensure that patients' and caregivers' needs are being met are suggested, such as enough time, a central contact person, an increasing focus on caregivers' needs, and widespread communication training. By integrating a theoretic basis of communication, empirical described needs, and practical suggestions for meeting these needs, this article hopes to provide an impetus for improved communication with seriously ill older people and their caregivers in uncertain and challenging times.

SUMMARY

This article aims to provide more insight into effective communication with older people with serious illness and their surrogates/caregivers. To do so, if focusses on specific skills in three core functions of communication (i) empathic behavior, (ii) information provision and (iii) enabling decision making. Empathy is always important and can be provided using 'NURSE', meanwhile assuring a continued relationship. As older people's abilities for information processing decreases, the importance of tailoring information is highlighted, using approaches as 'SPIKES' or 'Ask-tell-Ask' and providing chunks of information, while empathy also facilitates information processing. Eliciting patients' goals of care, with or without the help of surrogates, is important to come to effective decision making. Surrogates need assistance when making decisions for patients while they also have their own caregiver needs for support and information. Lastly, several suggestions to ensure patients' and caregivers' needs are being met are made, with the aim to improve communication in challenging and uncertain times.

ACKNOWLEDGMENTS

We thank the Dutch Cancer Society for their financial support of this article (for J.C.M. van Weert, PhD (grant number UVA 2010-4740)). The Dutch Cancer Society had no role in the study design, in the writing of the report, and in the decision to submit the article for publication.

REFERENCES

1. Morrison RS, Meier DE. Palliative care. N Engl J Med 2004;350:2582–90.
2. Ptacek JT, Ptacek JJ. Patients' perceptions of receiving bad news about cancer. J Clin Oncol 2001;19:4160–4.
3. Schofield P, Butow P, Thompson J, et al. Psychological responses of patients receiving a diagnosis of cancer. Ann Oncol 2003;14:48–56.
4. Jansen J, van Weert JC, de Groot J, et al. Emotional and informational patient cues: the impact of nurses' responses on recall. Patient Educ Couns 2010;79: 218–24.
5. van Osch M, Sep M, van Vliet LM, et al. Reducing patients' anxiety and uncertainty, and improving recall in bad news consultations. Health Psychol 2014;33: 1382–90.
6. Sep MS, van Osch M, van Vliet LM, et al. The power of clinicians' affective communication: how reassurance about non-abandonment can reduce patients' physiological arousal and increase information recall in bad news consultations. An experimental study using analogue patients. Patient Educ Couns 2014;95:45–52.
7. Wright AA, Zhang B, Ray A, et al. Associations between end-of-life discussions, patient mental health, medical care near death, and caregiver bereavement adjustment. JAMA 2008;300:1665–73.
8. Zhang B, Wright AA, Huskamp HA, et al. Health care costs in the last week of life: associations with end-of-life conversations. Arch Intern Med 2009;169:480–8.
9. de Haes H, Bensing J. Endpoints in medical communication research, proposing a framework of functions and outcomes. Patient Educ Couns 2009;74:287–94.
10. Bensing JM, Deveugele M, Moretti F, et al. How to make the medical consultation more successful from a patient's perspective? Tips for doctors and patients from lay people in the United Kingdom, Italy, Belgium and the Netherlands. Patient Educ Couns 2011;84:287–93.
11. Parker PA, Baile WF, de Moor C, et al. Breaking bad news about cancer: patients' preferences for communication. J Clin Oncol 2001;19:2049–56.
12. Belanger E, Rodriguez C, Groleau D. Shared decision-making in palliative care: a systematic mixed studies review using narrative synthesis. Palliat Med 2011;25: 242–61.
13. Parker SM, Clayton JM, Hancock K, et al. A systematic review of prognostic/end-of-life communication with adults in the advanced stages of a life-limiting illness: patient/caregiver preferences for the content, style, and timing of information. J Pain Symptom Manage 2007;34:81–93.

14. Puts MT, Papoutsis A, Springall E, et al. A systematic review of unmet needs of newly diagnosed older cancer patients undergoing active cancer treatment. Support Care Cancer 2012;20:1377–94.
15. Jansen J, van Weert J, van Dulmen S, et al. Patient education about treatment in cancer care. Cancer Nurs 2007;30:251–60.
16. Sparks L, O'Hair HD, Kreps GL. Cancer, communication and aging. New York: Hamptom Press, Inc; 2008.
17. Cai J, Clark J, Croft S, et al. Indications of Public Health in the English Regions. 9: Older People. York (UK): Alcuin Research and Resource Centre University of York; 2008.
18. Delgado-Guay MO, De La Cruz MG, Epner DE. 'I don't want to burden my family': handling communication challenges in geriatric oncology. Ann Oncol 2013; 24:30–5.
19. Sparks L, Nussbaum JF. Health literacy and cancer communication with older adults. Patient Educ Couns 2008;71:345–50.
20. Posma ER, van Weert JC, Jansen J, et al. Older cancer patients' information and support needs surrounding treatment: an evaluation through the eyes of patients, relatives and professionals. BMC Nurs 2009;8:1.
21. Jansen J, van Weert J, van der Meulen N, et al. Recall in older cancer patients: measuring memory for medical information. Gerontologist 2008;48:149–57.
22. Thorne S, Hislop TG, Kim-Sing C, et al. Changing communication needs and preferences across the cancer care trajectory: insights from the patient perspective. Support Care Cancer 2014;22:1009–15.
23. Fogarty LA, Curbow BA, Wingard JR, et al. Can 40 seconds of compassion reduce patient anxiety? J Clin Oncol 1999;17:371–9.
24. Back AL, Young JP, McCown E, et al. Abandonment at the end of life from patient, caregiver, nurse, and physician perspectives: loss of continuity and lack of closure. Arch Intern Med 2009;169:474–9.
25. van Vliet LM, van der Wall E, Plum NM, et al. Explicit prognostic information and reassurance about nonabandonment when entering palliative breast cancer care: findings from a scripted video-vignette study. J Clin Oncol 2013;31:3242–9.
26. Back AL, Arnold RM, Baile WF, et al. Approaching difficult communication tasks in oncology. CA Cancer J Clin 2005;55:164–77.
27. Smith RC, Hoppe RB. The patient's story: integrating the patient-and physician-centered approaches to interviewing. Ann Intern Med 1991;115:470–7.
28. van Vliet LM, Epstein AS. Current state of the art and science of patient-clinician communication in progressive disease: patients' need to know and need to feel known. J Clin Oncol 2014;32:3474–8.
29. Bruera E, Palmer JL, Pace E, et al. A randomized, controlled trial of physician postures when breaking bad news to cancer patients. J Palliat Med 2007; 21:501–5.
30. Bolle S, Muusses LD, Smets EM, et al. Chemotherapie, wat weet u er van? Een onderzoek naar de publieke kennis, perceptie van bijwerkingen, informatiebehoeften en het gebruik van informatiebronnen met betrekking tot chemotherapie. [Chemotherapy, what do you know about it. A national study into public knowledge, perception of side effects, information needs and the use of information sources about chemotherapy]. Amsterdam: Amsterdam School of Communication Research/ASCoR, Universiteit van Amsterdam; 2012.
31. van Weert J, Bolle S, van Dulmen S, et al. Older cancer patients' information and communication needs: what they want is what they get? Patient Educ Couns 2013;92:388–97.

32. Mather M, Carstensen LL. Aging and motivated cognition: the positivity effect in attention and memory. Trends Cogn Sci 2005;9:496–502.
33. Peters E, Hibbard J, Slovic P, et al. Numeracy skill and the communication, comprehension, and use of risk-benefit information. Health Aff (Millwood) 2007; 26:741–8.
34. Brown SC, Park DC. Theoretical models of cognitive aging and implications for translational research in medicine. Gerontologist 2003;43:57–67.
35. Salthouse TA. The nature of the influence of speed on adult age-differences in cognition. Dev Psychol 1994;30:240–59.
36. Bopp KL, Verhaeghen P. Aging and verbal memory span: a meta-analysis. J Gerontol B Psychol Sci Soc Sci 2005;60:223–33.
37. Amieva H, Phillips L, Della Sala S. Behavioral dysexecutive symptoms in normal aging. Brain Cogn 2003;53:129–32.
38. Baile WF, Buckman R, Lenzi R, et al. SPIKES—a six-step protocol for delivering bad news: application to the patient with cancer. Oncologist 2000;5:302–11.
39. Brom L, Hopmans W, Pasman HR, et al. Congruence between patients' preferred and perceived participation in medical decision-making: a review of the literature. BMC Med Inform Decis Mak 2014;14:25.
40. Edwards A, Elwyn G. Inside the black box of shared decision making: distinguishing between the process of involvement and who makes the decision. Health Expect 2006;9:307–20.
41. LeBlanc A, Kenny DA, O'Connor AM, et al. Decisional conflict in patients and their physicians: a dyadic approach to shared decision making. Med Decis Making 2009;29:61–8.
42. Stacey D, Bennett CL, Barry MJ, et al. Decision aids for people facing health treatment or screening decisions. Cochrane Database Syst Rev 2011;(10): CD001431.
43. Stiggelbout AM, Van der Weijden T, De Wit MP, et al. Shared decision making: really putting patients at the centre of healthcare. BMJ 2012;344:e256.
44. McCaffery KJ, Holmes-Rovner M, Smith SK, et al. Addressing health literacy in patient decision aids. BMC Med Inform Decis Mak 2013;13:S10.
45. Lee CN, Chang YC, Adimorah N, et al. Decision making about surgery for early-stage breast cancer. J Am Coll Surg 2012;214:1–10.
46. Steinhauser KE, Christakis NA, Clipp EC, et al. Factors considered important at the end of life by patients, family, physicians, and other care providers. JAMA 2000;284:2476–82.
47. Quill T, Norton S, Shah M, et al. What is most important for you to achieve?: an analysis of patient responses when receiving palliative care consultation. J Palliat Med 2006;9:382–8.
48. Back AL, Arnold RM, Quill TE. Hope for the best, and prepare for the worst. Ann Intern Med 2003;138:439–43.
49. Mata R, Schooler LJ, Rieskamp J. The aging decision maker: cognitive aging and the adaptive selection of decision strategies. Psychol Aging 2007;22: 796–810.
50. Reed AE, Mikels JA, Simon KI. Older adults prefer less choice than young adults. Psychol Aging 2008;23:671–5.
51. Finucane ML, Mertz CK, Slovic P, et al. Task complexity and older adults' decision-making competence. Psychol Aging 2005;20:71–84.
52. Allen MS, Darling GE, Pechet TT, et al. Morbidity and mortality of major pulmonary resections in patients with early-stage lung cancer: initial results of the randomized, prospective ACOSOG Z0030 trial. Ann Thorac Surg 2006;81:1013–20.

53. Scott IA, Guyatt GH. Cautionary tales in the interpretation of clinical studies involving older persons. Arch Intern Med 2010;170:587–95.
54. Sessums LL, Zembrzuska H, Jackson JL. Does this patient have medical decision-making capacity? JAMA 2011;306:420–7.
55. Torke AM, Sachs GA, Helft PR, et al. Scope and outcomes of surrogate decision making among hospitalized older adults. JAMA Intern Med 2014;174:370–7.
56. Schenker Y, Crowley-Matoka M, Dohan D, et al. I don't want to be the one saying 'we should just let him die': intrapersonal tensions experienced by surrogate decision makers in the ICU. J Gen Intern Med 2012;27:1657–65.
57. Quill TE, Arnold R, Back AL. Discussing treatment preferences with patients who want "everything". Ann Intern Med 2009;151:345–9.
58. Andershed B. Relatives in end-of-life care–part 1: a systematic review of the literature the five last years, January 1999–February 2004. J Clin Nurs 2006;15: 1158–69.
59. Powazki R, Walsh D, Hauser K, et al. Communication in palliative medicine: a clinical review of family conferences. J Palliat Med 2014;17:1167–77.
60. Hudson P, Remedios C, Zordan R, et al. Guidelines for the psychosocial and bereavement support of family caregivers of palliative care patients. J Palliat Med 2012;15:696–702.
61. Salthouse TA. Why do adult age-differences increase with task complexity. Dev Psychol 1992;28:905–18.

Communications by Professionals in Palliative Care

Lidia Schapira, MD

KEYWORDS

- Geriatric • Palliative care • Clinical practice • Communication • Caregiver
- Family ageism • Uncertainty • End of life

KEY POINTS

- Involve family caregivers in decision making, as this enables them to make plans and complete advance directives that conform to their values and preferences.
- Family meetings are useful during transitions in care; addressing the emotions and fears of family members through empathic connections and strategies may improve outcomes.
- Recognize ageist bias.
- Assist patients to share what matters most before discussing advance directives.

INTRODUCTION

Good communication is at the core of palliative care, providing a medium for clinicians to express their concern and respect for patients that honors the mission of medicine. The patients' humanity evokes feelings of solidarity and empathy that lead to the compassionate care we all want for ourselves and for those we love. The moral aspects of caring become apparent in the guidance we provide and also in the choices patients and their loved ones make every day. Fluid communication allows clinicians to inform patients and to receive valuable information in return. Thus, communication skills are essential for responding to challenging clinical situations, providing leadership to a multidisciplinary team, and supporting trainees.

Although there is a robust literature on clinician-patient communication, clinical practice is derived from observed practices and consensus-driven guidelines. Many such guidelines were formulated with young or middle-aged patients in mind, individuals who prefer to act autonomously and who are interested in sharing the responsibility of medical decisions with professionals. Research has focused on

The author has no disclosures to report or conflicts of interest and she is the sole author of this article.

Massachusetts General Hospital, Department of Hematology-Oncology, 55 Fruit Street, Yawkey 9-A, Boston, MA 02114, USA

E-mail address: lschapira@partners.org

how best to inform those patients who still think of their future in very broad terms, imagining they have decades left to live, but fail to capture the pressing concerns of the very old. It seems reasonable that middle-aged patients may consider present tradeoffs for the sake of future gains, whereas older individuals may prefer not to sacrifice their independence or present quality of life for the possibility of a short extension of their life. These differences in outlook and perspective add another layer of complexity and need to be taken into consideration.

Excellent communication conveys a powerful message of service and compassion to patients and their families and helps to establish collegial relationships among members of a multidisciplinary team. Cultivating these skills is essential in order to broach difficult topics and to help patients and their families articulate their preferences for care when confronted with complex treatment options or when they transition to end-of-life care. Communication can be just as powerful as any drug and needs to be carefully dosed and tailored to meet the needs of individual patients. Meaningful conversations can enable patients and family caregivers to make plans and complete advance directives that conform to their values and preferences. Engaging patients and families in the process of completing advance directives and designating a health care proxy is an important step toward closing the gap between those who say they hope to spend their final days at home and the small proportion that actually do.

In 2009, approximately 1 in 4 adults aged 65 years and older died in acute care hospitals, 1 in 3 in nursing homes, and 1 in 3 at home.[1,2] Among all decedents, 1 in 3 experienced an admission to the intensive care unit (ICU) in the month preceding death. A recent report by the Institute of Medicine, *Dying in America*, provides convincing data that too many older individuals die in overmedicalized environments because they were unprepared to make important decisions that could have helped them maintain a semblance of control and dignity in the final weeks and months. The report is a call to action, clearly noting that there is an urgent need to engage older patients and their family caregivers in frank conversations about death and dying and to coach them to think about their preferences for care during the final weeks or months. Furthermore, given our inability to predict the final weeks or months of life, it is imperative that these matters are discussed before the illness becomes advanced.

In this article, the author first examines the ageist bias that is prevalent in clinics today and then reviews the basic communication principles and strategies that can help clinicians make their conversations with patients more focused and meaningful, thereby preparing patients and their family caregivers to make decisions in a crisis and to engage in planning for end-of-life care as early and intensively as possible.

AGEISM

Adults worry that as they grow older, they will be less able to fully enjoy the world. New research has begun to emerge showing that the opposite is true; in fact, when adults of all ages are asked about their sense of well-being, the oldest group tends to respond more positively than other age groups. In a new and optimistic book on aging, Holland and Greenstein[3] posit that well-being is in the shape of a U: high during young adulthood dropping to its lowest around 50 years of age then rebounding and rising continuously. Stanford Psychologist Laura Carstensen[4] suggests that with age comes greater motivation to find a sense of meaning in life and less of a need to focus on expanding personal horizons. This mindset allows for more thoughtful decision-making when it comes to life or economic choices.[4,5] Unfortunately, we know very little about how the old and very old make important medical decisions; despite this new optimism surrounding healthy aging and the benefits of longevity, health care professionals sometimes harbor implicit biases about older individuals that interfere with their assessments and practice.

Young physicians are exposed to the most vulnerable among the hospitalized elderly: those who are frail and perhaps cognitively impaired or socially isolated. Young clinicians may experience anxiety and fear obsolescence and death, and, without the ability to process and work through these issues, may develop ageist attitudes that interfere with their judgment. We know that physicians are less likely to recommend prevention practices without the requisite deliberation based on life expectancy and the patients' preference. Physicians also misattribute or dismiss symptoms as normal aging when the symptom profile merits a work-up and could indicate a treatable condition.

Katherine Graham, former publisher of the *Washington Post*, was still running her company and skiing into her eighties, whereas other octogenarians require assistance to perform the basic activities of daily living, such as bathing and feeding. Geriatric assessments eliminate guesswork and provide validated and useful estimates of function across multiple domains that help guide clinical decision making.[6] Common deficits associated with aging include decreases in hearing and vision as well as subtle cognitive dysfunction. If a patient is hard of hearing, take the time to position yourself so that he or she can hear you. Even if the patient has mild cognitive dysfunction, he or she may still be able to choose a course of treatment. Older individuals may also be more limited in terms of their financial resources and social support, defined as a network of close relatives and friends who can potentially help a patient during an illness.[7] Social support likely enables older patients who need some form of assistance to attend clinic appointments, undergo diagnostic testing, receive treatments for their illnesses, and to feel emotionally sustained.

When it comes to communication, the most important clinical difference between younger and more elderly patients is that important conversations with older patients often involve a third party, typically a spouse or adult child. There has been little research to date about the complexities of a 3- or 4-way conversation, but it is essential to acknowledge the presence and needs of that third party. After all, it is often this individual who will assume the important role of patient advocate and voice the patients' preferences during unforeseen crises leading to hospitalizations.

THE FOCUSED CONVERSATION

Illness is an isolating experience, and patients may defer difficult talks about the future. We need to consider the natural reluctance of patients and their families to open the conversation and explore not only their reasons for avoidance but also our own as clinicians (**Box 1**). The reality is that most patients who die in hospitals are under the care of doctors who never knew them when they were well.[2] In the absence of an advance care plan, patients and their families struggle with decisions that feel abrupt and for which they are not well prepared. We should think of advance care planning not as a one-time activity but, instead, as a series of profound and focused conversations about life and what matters most.

What patients understand or misunderstand about the course of their illness can affect the treatment decisions they make.[8,9] Our professional culture expects that, as clinicians, we will do everything possible to extend life as long as it is meaningful for the patients. Our society at large expects that patients will fight disease and honor those who fight until they take their last breath, without paying sufficient attention to

---

Box 1
Communication is a diagnostic and therapeutic tool

The intern is paged to the surgical floor at 5 AM to evaluate an 84-year-old woman 2 days after a hip replacement. She pulled out her intravenous line and is trying to get out of bed. Yesterday she seemed fine and had a nice visit with her family. Today she is disoriented and combative, and the nursing staff is considering the use of restraints. After assessing the situation, the young physician recognizes the patient is delirious and consults the palliative care team. She feels overwhelmed when the patient's family approaches her and asks her what is going on.

The palliative care consultant takes a detailed history from the patient's family and nursing staff, reviews the medication list and recent laboratory studies, looks at the overall time course, performs a limited mental status examination, and confirms the diagnosis of delirium. He meets with the team and recommends a combination of pharmacologic and nonpharmacologic interventions that take into consideration the patient's age and risk of harm. He is careful to involve the family in the plan and encourages the nursing staff to work collaboratively with the family to reorient and reassure the patient. He then addresses the communication challenges with the intern and medical team. Here are the salient teaching points:

- Involving family caregivers provides an opportunity for the family and the medical team to share their understanding and worries about care and to solidify a therapeutic relationship.
- Communication is a 2-way street for information exchange, and the patient will benefit if the family is invited to participate in team discussions, perhaps providing crucial information, such as the use of as-needed medications at home or a history of substance abuse.
- Use circular questions to explore the family's concerns: *What worries you the most?*
- Use strategic and focused questions to obtain information: *What medications did your mother take the day before she was admitted to the hospital?*
- Provide a wrap-up that is clear to the family, avoids jargon, and gives them a working narrative that they can share and understand: *This is temporary and caused by the medications she received during and after surgery and will get better in a matter of a few days. It would be very helpful if you or your sister could stay by her bedside and help us orient her and keep her safe.*

---

the price exacted from those who insist on aggressive and often futile treatment toward the end of life. Patients may have insufficient knowledge regarding medical interventions, such as cardiopulmonary resuscitation (CPR), and may be unduly influenced by the media or depictions of heroic measures stemming from the entertainment industry.[10] If patients do not ask questions, doctors may think that patients know as much as they need, or want, to know. A productive working relationship between a doctor and patient requires that the doctor understand that individual patient's needs, goals, and expectations of care and the responsibility for arriving at that understanding must be shared between them.

The older people are, the more likely they are to have participated in some kind of advanced planning activity. People of means are more likely to engage in estate and financial planning, an activity that can trigger some aspects of health-related planning, such as establishing a durable power of attorney.[11] A California survey asked adults of all ages whether they had spoken with a loved one about their wishes for end-of-life medical treatment. Among those who had not, the most important reasons were the following: "don't want to think about it" or "family members don't want to discuss."[12] As clinicians, we deal with the consequences of patients' unwillingness to discuss these matters; when these conversations actually do take place, and lead to the completion of an advance directive, the document is often misplaced or unavailable at a time of need. A recent study showed that completed advance directives were missing in half of the charts of patients older than 75 years of age.[13]

Providing clear information, avoiding jargon, and pausing frequently constitutes a good delivery but is no guarantee that patients actually understood the information. If you recognize that patients did not understand you, rephrase your statement instead of repeating or speaking louder. Patients retain only a fraction of the information they are given; when the news is bad, they often distort the message perhaps as a defense mechanism. Paying attention to emotional cues through gentle exploration and providing strong assurance of nonabandonment, such as saying *I am willing to be here with you*, will allow patients to begin to process the information.[14–16] It is better to think of advance care planning as a multistep and iterative process rather than a menu offering different but equally undesirable options.

Well-meaning professionals often exaggerate the harm caused by potentially futile medical procedures in order to be more persuasive. Studies have convincingly shown that visual aids, including video, can be helpful to patients by providing information about specific interventions, such as CPR.[10] Patients described these tools as helpful and felt comfortable watching them, and those who did watch the video gained a more realistic view of their options along with the accompanying risks and benefits.[10] Ideally these visual aids should be paired with a debriefing conversation with a clinician, thus giving patients a chance to reflect and check their understanding before addressing their preferences and choices.

A technique that never fails is to focus on life and living rather than death and dying (**Box 2**). If clinicians first ask themselves who the patients are and what matters most to them, it is more likely that they will relax and see patients as people and allow them to convey important information about what gives their life meaning or purpose. Their life may revolve around their dog, their family, a volunteer activity, or their faith. Watching for signs of pride or recognition helps clinicians to identify the themes in the patients' narratives that are important and then weave them into their focused discussion in a way that helps the patients feel known. Clinicians can prepare patients and surrogates to make the best possible in-the-moment medical decisions by gently

---

Box 2
Three questions

Ron Sabar is an Israeli physician who leads teams that deliver home hospice care. They treat 2000 patients per year, with a 100% death rate and almost 100% satisfaction from patients and their families. In a recent TED talk in Jerusalem in 2014, he shared some of his insights.

Sabar reminded the audience that most of us will not die a sudden death. Instead, we will be aware of the fact that we are dying and will die a slow and progressive death. This circumstance allows us the privilege of maintaining some level of dignity and control and that, in and of itself, is a source of meaning and self-worth. Sabar acknowledges that talking about death and dying is difficult. He offers a small gift based on his lived experience, and this consists of 3 questions that open conversations:

1. *What do you understand about your condition?* It may be the first time families realize patients actually know their prognosis and may provide an opportunity to discuss plans for the future.

2. *What you are most afraid of?* Most patients respond that they are afraid of suffering, of being in pain, of becoming a burden, or dying alone.

3. *What would make you happy now?* Sabar's patients typically offer tangible and durable responses that speak of immediate and realizable goals, such as talking to my sister, seeing the house I helped design, or attending a family wedding.

exploring their understanding of, and attitudes toward, death.[17] During routine visits, a clinician can ask patients if they are avoiding the conversation about their illness and then identify the reasons for avoidance. Perhaps patients wish to protect a loved one or fear becoming a burden. For those who prefer to avoid an emotionally laden conversation, a useful approach is to focus on the goals of care.

Communication Tips
- If a patient is hard of hearing, take the time to position yourself so that he or she can hear you.
- If you recognize the patient did not understand you, rephrase your statement (do not repeat).
- If a patient has mild cognitive impairment, he or she may still be able to make medical decisions.
- If there are both family and paid caregivers, recognize them and address their roles and needs.
- If you struggle with the emotional content of a conversation, focus on the goals and wishes.

SHARING UNCERTAINTY

Uncertainty is often triggered by hearing bad news, by an unplanned hospitalization, or meeting a new doctor. Not knowing is unsettling, not only for patients but also for the doctor. A common theme in narratives of illness and suffering is that patients want to be known and respected by their professional caregivers. Another is that relationships matter and have a healing quality, even in the face of therapeutic failure.[18] Patients are concerned with relationships and are comforted by explicit statements of nonabandonment; they appreciate when doctors acknowledge their difficulties and offer to share the task of making important decisions.[14–16,19] Some patients may experience uncertainty as a traumatic event or a threat and harbor complex feelings, including disappointment, frustration, anger, and shock. They need guidance and a safe space to come to terms with the disruption in their lives and restore a sense of coherence to their personal narrative.[20] In the context of a long patient-clinician relationship, the physician can sometimes model how she or he deals with not knowing and create a shared experience and, through this therapeutic engagement, propel patients to find their own way of coping with adversity. A frequently taught and useful communication strategy is to help patients articulate worst- and best-case scenarios and then recommend planning for the worst while hoping for a better outcome.[21]

News of an unfavorable response to treatment or worsening of a chronic illness alters a person's relationship to the future. Some patients may find it difficult to verbalize thoughts or express sadness and may need a gentle nudge from skilled clinicians to help them understand the full impact of the news, especially if it necessitates a fundamental change in the medical plan, such as a transition from disease-modifying therapy to hospice care. Common communication pitfalls are to rush to reassure without giving patients the space and time to process their feelings or making wrongful assumptions about the patients' state of mind. Being married is no guarantee that patients feel supported or accompanied, and having ample financial resources does not protect a person from feeling helpless when facing the complex medical system; only detailed inquiry provides a complete picture of the individual patient's coping and available supports.

A simple model that helps facilitate these difficult conversations is to imagine the bad news as an existential threat that feels chaotic and to pace the therapeutic encounter so that patients have a chance to understand and experience the consequences of such news. On coming to terms with the threat, the clinician can help patients transform that threat into a challenge. Asking someone to reconfigure their aspirations or hopes for the future can be daunting and requires imagination, time, inner strength, and support. Helping patients to reframe their hopes and expectations after learning they have limited time or diminished capacity remains one of the most challenging aspects of palliative care medicine.

WHAT LIES AHEAD?

In July 1982, Stephen Jay Gould, an American biologist, paleontologist, and historian of science, was diagnosed with peritoneal mesothelioma. Two years later, Gould[22] published a column for *Discover Magazine* entitled "The Median Isn't the Message," which discusses his reaction to discovering that patients with mesothelioma had a median lifespan of only 8 months after diagnosis.[22] He describes the true significance behind this number and his relief on realizing that statistical averages are just useful abstractions and do not encompass the full range of variation. To be more specific, he calculated he should be in the favorable half of the upper statistical range because he was young, the disease was diagnosed early, and he had access to cutting-edge therapies. He enrolled in a clinical trial and was also treated with radiation and surgery. He lived 20 years free of cancer and died of a second malignancy.

Unlike Professor Gould, older patients typically find themselves in the unfavorable half of the lower statistical range. Treatments for advanced stages of most chronic illnesses are tolerated poorly, and the tradeoffs implicit in choosing between extending life or losing one's independence can be heartbreaking. On a positive note, older patients can be more accepting that life has to end and more invested in ending their lives without becoming a burden to others or prolonging the dying process. Older patients may worry about depleting their financial resources or needing to be institutionalized in the final months and many have had plenty of experience watching relatives or friends who struggled with the same choices.

After Gould's essay and for the next 3 decades, physicians struggled to improve the accuracy and precision of their prognoses. The work of Lamont and Christakis[23] showed that physicians consistently overestimate a patient's life expectancy in the setting of an advanced illness, up to a factor of 5. Moreover Christakis[24] argued convincingly that physicians have a moral responsibility or duty to inform patients and must convey a realistic time frame or prognosis in order to help patients make informed choices. Medical educators, researchers, and experienced clinicians focused on providing practical tips to improve the delivery of bad news and prognostic estimates through sample scripts and visual aids in order to simplify the message contained in mathematical constructs of means, medians, and averages.[25–27] Studies confirmed what clinicians suspected: most patients prefer to receive honest and timely information, even when the prognosis is bad.[28] And yet audiotaped conversations between patients with hematologic malignancies and their consultants showed that more than 20% of patients recalled a different estimate of survival from what was originally offered by the doctor.[29] This information serves as a powerful reminder that individual patients may not be able to hear bad news and use denial as a protective mechanism if they are overwhelmed.[30,31]

Discussions of prognosis should go beyond estimates of life expectancy and include information about the likely evolution of the disease. It may take repeated conversations over many weeks or months for a person to be able to process the information. Patients often express ambivalence about receiving any news that is not favorable, and clinicians may choose to defer such conversations while the disease seems to be stable. Gould's wisdom can serve to remind us that the median is not the message and that conveying prognostic information is one of the most challenging tasks for clinicians dealing with patients who are seriously ill.

INVOLVING THE FAMILY

A patient's experience of illness cannot be understood in isolation from his or her family and environment. Clinicians need to appreciate a patient's beliefs and the central role of family caregivers. Resilient families rally during a crisis and patients come to depend on spouses or adult children to make fundamental choices that are concordant with their values and informed by lived experiences. Dysfunctional families may not be able to agree on a course of action, and the tension generated by divergent viewpoints or expectations may require expert mediation.

Family is defined as the network of friends, relatives, neighbors and congregants who assume shared responsibility for caregiving outside of a hospital or nursing home environment. Although, in past times, women were widely expected to assume the role of the caregiver, today's families are smaller, and more women have paid jobs outside the home. Care is often quite complex and involves physical tasks, such as managing stomas and catheters, administering medications, coordinating appointments, and communicating with health care professionals. About half of adults with regular jobs also spend more than 3 years in a care-giving role.[2] It is estimated that a staggering $25 billion are lost annually through diminished productivity because of absenteeism caused by family caregiving.[2] For frail elders and patients with advanced illness, many of whom may have multiple chronic diseases, patient-centered care is impossible to imagine without caregiver; the caregiver's contribution to end-of-life care and planning deserves more attention.

After-death interviews with 205 families of adult decedents included several questions related to advance care planning. Higher scores were associated with communication about treatment preferences, compliance with treatment preferences, and family satisfaction regarding communication with clinical staff.[32] Specific aspects of the communication that were surveyed included how well the professional team listened to the family, how well they explained the condition in language the family members could understand, and whether the clinicians used terms that were meaningful to the family members.[32]

Patients who are reluctant to complete advance directives may benefit from hearing personal stories of others who have had to make end-of-life decisions for a loved one without any guidance. Ultimately the desire to save one's family from these painful experiences can become a prime motivator for putting these wishes in writing.[2,33,34] One study found that 70% of decedents aged 60 years or older participating in a longitudinal study of health and retirement were incapable of participating in conversations about their treatment in the final phase of life.[2,35] Involving family caregivers is a crucial step in mobilizing patients.[36] Research studies have shed light on the fact that family caregivers are at risk for anxiety and depression as a result of perceived burdens of caregiving and that it is important to encourage caregivers to pay attention to their own needs and self-care.[37] Little is known about the factors that make caregivers more or less accurate as surrogate decision makers for their loved ones. Cartensen and colleagues[38] found that attachment orientation influences the likelihood that adult children (and other relatives) know their parents' end-of-life health care wishes.

Palliative care professionals can help patients and families overcome their reticence and engage in conversations that will prepare them to make informed choices about their care. This process begins with a gentle exploration of their prognostic awareness, their expectations and hopes for recovery, and their readiness to talk about the final separation. With a third person in the room to guide them and contain the affect, spouses or parents and children are often able to say to each other what they may otherwise keep to themselves.

FACILITATING A FAMILY MEETING

Patients and their families are often asked to make difficult decisions without much warning and without sufficient understanding of their choices. Hospital routines are anything but restful, and care is often experienced as fragmented with assignments to teams of strangers that change every shift. Patients or their health care proxy may harbor unrealistic expectations about recovery, sometimes as a result of inborn optimism but more often because they have not heard clear and consistent information from professionals they know and trust. Although we embrace teamwork, this team approach may have the unintended consequence of making patients feel abandoned because they no longer have one primary doctor. Palliative care clinicians often find patients and families are confused about the news they received and need to sort out the relevant aspects of the case.

In hospital settings and especially in the ICU, a family meeting provides a mechanism for the exchange of vital information and assists patients and their families at times of transitions in care. Patients may be too ill to participate; spouses may be in shock; and adult children may be suffering from confusing emotions, including guilt and sadness. Addressing the emotions and fears of family members through empathic connections and strategies may improve outcomes, such as reducing psychological symptoms of trauma, anxiety, and depression; shortening ICU length of stay; and improving the experience of dying.[39,40]

There is a paucity of research about family conferences; most studies are narrative, observational, or qualitative. Rhondali and colleagues[41] surveyed palliative care representatives from all registered palliative care units (PCUs) in the French National Association for Palliative Care database (N = 113). Questionnaires were sent to all directors of PCUs with a request to forward them to the palliative care physician in charge of the unit, the nurse, the psychologist, and the social worker (n = 452). With a 61% response rate from 81% of units, they found that only 5% reported following a structured protocol. The 3 primary goals of family conferences were to allow family members to express their feelings, to identify family caregivers, and discuss the patients' plan of care. The primary reasons for conducting a family conference were (1) a terminal illness, (2) family caregivers' request, or (3) terminal sedation required. Thirty-eight percent reported that patients were not invited to participate. The primary indications and goals were significantly different among the 4 health care disciplines. In general, the goals of the physicians, social workers, nurses, and psychologists were consistent with their professional contexts and backgrounds. For instance, physicians discussed refractory symptoms, and social workers commented on the need to identify the primary family caregiver. One of the surprising results was the very low percentage of palliative care professionals who preferred to conduct family conferences with patients participating in the full meeting (17%). These professionals cited concerns that patients are often delirious or that the patients' presence might block or inhibit the emotional expression of caregivers as explanations for their reluctance to include the patients in the meetings. Many expressed a preference for partial participation, a finding that is concordant with a US study.[42]

Experts recommend convening a preconference team meeting in order to set an agenda and to ensure that the clinicians who will participate really understand the medical and social situation, the important sources of potential distress, and the available options for patients and their families. Identifying who needs to be present is vital to a successful meeting, and this depends on understanding who patients identify as kin. Cofacilitation between a physician and social worker, for example, allows more even weighting of medical and psychosocial issues. As the meeting gets going past introductions, it is useful to explore the understanding of various members present and to ask a few questions to probe their coping style and resiliency. For instance asking how they have dealt with prior family crises may help you evaluate how this family may or may not be able to reorganize roles, rules, and ways of relating to each other in order to care for the ill member and to support one another. Resilient families impress us every day with resourceful solutions, flexibility, and endurance during difficult times. On the other hand, dysfunctional families have a very limited ability to function as a team, as individual relatives are less involved and may not regularly communicate with each other or may be openly hostile. They may come across as argumentative, and it is important to note that they are at risk for complicated bereavement.

The facilitators need to maintain a compassionate stance and ask clarifying questions in order to make family members feel welcome and at ease. If clinicians leading the meeting have a preexisting relationship with the patients and families, they can remind the families of prior important events or decisions they made together.[43] If there is no joint history, clinicians need to build immediate rapport and ask directly about the patients' prior thoughts about living and dying, such as the following: *Did your father talk about where he would want to die? Did you and your mother talk about her feelings of being kept alive by machines in an intensive care unit? If the patient could speak to us right now, how might he or she guide us in our decision making?* When physicians use words such as death and dying rather than euphemisms, the conversation is more authentic. When patients hear doctors talk about withholding potentially life-saving interventions, they may feel conflicted or guilty. Choosing words and expressions that convey a more peaceful image, such as *allowing natural death*, may help dispel the tension.

Family meetings allow caregivers to ask for support and to learn more about their options both in terms of available medical treatments as well as services that can be rendered in the community following discharge from the hospital. These meetings allow discussion of caregiving roles and the liaison with medical teams and guide families to make decisions by consensus. Palliative care clinicians can assist families in solving practical problems, such as arranging for home services, and also provide a forum for discussion of complex dilemmas that often encompass spiritual and religious concerns.

SUMMARY

As longevity becomes more common and we get better at controlling chronic diseases, such as heart failure or cancer, it is easy to be lulled into the belief that death may be postponed or avoided.[2] Patients, family caregivers, and clinicians often avoid having conversations about difficult issues, such as death and dying. The consequence is that when the illness cannot be controlled, patients and family caregivers may be unprepared to make tough choices about treatment; this leads to unwanted and futile care, greater psychological distress, and complicated bereavement.

Palliative care clinicians are committed to family-centered care that is concordant with patients' beliefs and worldview with the ultimate goal of reducing suffering in all its domains. Communication can serve both as medium and tool to explore concerns and provide solace and has extraordinary therapeutic potential. Cultivating communication skills through reflection, observation, skills training, and practice is a lifelong process and patients are our best teachers.

REFERENCES

1. Teno JM, Gozalo PL, Bynum JP, et al. Change in end-of –life care for Medicare beneficiaries: site of death, place of care, and health care transitions in 2000, 2005 and 2009. JAMA 2013;309(5):470–7.
2. IOM (Institute of Medicine). Dying in America. Washington, DC: National Academy Press; 2014.
3. Greenstein M, Holland J. Lighter as we go. Virtues, character strengths, and aging. New York: Oxford University Press; 2015.
4. Carstensen L. Our aging population. In: Irving P, editor. The upside of aging. Hoboken (NJ): John Wiley and Sons; 2014.
5. Mikels JA, Lockenhoff CE, Maglio SJ, et al. Following your heard or your head: focusing on emotions versus information differentially influences the decisions of younger and older adults. J Exp Psychol Appl 2010;16(1):87–95.
6. Wildiers H, Heeren P, Puts M, et al. International Society of Geriatric Oncology consensus on geriatric assessment in older patients with cancer. J Clin Oncol 2014;32:2595–603.
7. Sjolander C, Ahlstrom G. The meaning and validation of social support networks for close family of persons with advanced cancer. BMC Nurs 2012;11:17.
8. Weeks JC, Catalano PJ, Cronin A, et al. Patients' expectations about effects of chemotherapy for advanced cancer. N Engl J Med 2012;367:1616–25.
9. Smith TJ, Longo DL. Talking with patients about dying. N Engl J Med 2012;367: 1651–2.
10. Volandes AE, Paasche-Orlow MK, Mitchell SL. Randomized controlled trial of a video decision support tool for cardiopulmonary resuscitation decision making in advanced cancer. J Clin Oncol 2013;31(3):380–6.
11. Carr D. The social stratification of older adults' preparations for end-of-life healthcare. J Health Soc Behav 2012;53(3):297–312.
12. CHCF (California HealthCare Foundation). Final chapter. Californians' attitudes and experiences with death and dying. 2012. Available at: http://www.chcf.org/publications/2012/final-chapter-death-dying. Accessed October 18, 2014.
13. Yung VY, Walling AM, Min L. Documentation of advance care planning for community-dwelling elders. J Palliat Med 2010;13(7):861–7.
14. Van Vliet LM, van der Wall E, Plum NM, et al. Explicit prognostic information and reassurance about nonabandonment when entering palliative breast cancer care: findings from a scripted video-vignette study. J Clin Oncol 2013;31:3242–9.
15. Quill TE, Cassel CK. Nonabandonment: a central obligation for physicians. Ann Intern Med 1995;122:368–74.
16. Back A, Young JP, McCown E, et al. Abandonment at the end of life from patient, caregiver, nurse and physician perspectives: loss of continuity and lack of closure. Arch Intern Med 2009;169:474–9.
17. Sudore RL, Fried TR. Redefining the 'planning' in advance care planning: preparing for end-of-life decision-making. Ann Intern Med 2010;154(4):256–61.
18. Schapira L. Shared uncertainty. J Support Oncol 2004;2(1):14–8.

19. Salander P. Bad news from the patient's perspective: an analysis of the written narratives of newly diagnosed cancer patients. Soc Sci Med 2002;55:721–32.
20. Chochinov HM, McClement SE, Hack TH, et al. Healthcare provider communication: an empirical model of optimal therapeutic effectiveness. Cancer 2013;119:1706–13.
21. Back AL, Arnold RM, Quill TE. Hope for the best, and prepare for the worst. Ann Intern Med 2003;138:439–43.
22. Gould SJ. The median isn't the message. Discover 1985;6:40–2.
23. Lamont EB, Christakis N. Prognostic disclosure to patients with cancer near the end of life. Ann Intern Med 2001;134:1096–105.
24. Christakis N. Death foretold: prophecy and prognosis in medical care. Chicago: University of Chicago Press; 1999.
25. Baile WF, Buckman R, Lenzi R, et al. SPIKES: a six-step protocol for delivering bad news – application to the patient with cancer. Oncologist 2000;5:302–11.
26. Clayton JM, Hancock K, Butow PN. Clinical practice guidelines for communicating prognosis and end-of-life issues with adults in the advanced stages of a life-limiting illness, and their caregivers. Med J Aust 2007;186(Suppl 12):S77.
27. Kiely BE, Martin AJ, Tattesall MH, et al. The median informs the message: accuracy of individualized scenarios for survival time based on oncologists' estimates. J Clin Oncol 2013;31(28):3565–71.
28. Mack JW, Cronin A, Taback N, et al. End-of-life care discussions among patients with advanced cancer: a cohort study. Ann Intern Med 2012;156(3):204–10.
29. Alexander SC, Sullivan AM, Back AL, et al. Information giving and receiving in hematological malignancy consultations. Psychooncology 2012;21(3):297–306.
30. Jackson VA, Jacobsen J, Greer J, et al. The cultivation of prognostic awareness through the provision of early palliative care in the ambulatory setting: a communication guide. J Palliat Med 2013;16(8):894–900.
31. Weissman A. The vulnerable self: confronting the ultimate questions insight books. New York: Plenum Press; 1993.
32. Curtis JR, Patrick DL, Engelberg RA, et al. A measure of the quality of dying and death. Initial validation using after-death interviews with family members. J Pain Symptom Manage 2002;24(1):117–31.
33. Halpern S. Shaping end-of-life care: behavioral economics and advance directives. Semin Respir Crit Care Med 2012;33(4):393–400.
34. Steinhauser KE, Christakis NA, Clipp EC. Factors considered important at the end of life by patients, family, physicians, and other care providers. JAMA 2000;284(19):2746–82.
35. Silveira MJ, Kim SY, Langa KM. Advance directives and outcomes of surrogate decision making before death. N Engl J Med 2010;362(13):1211–8.
36. Gillick MR. The critical role of family caregivers in achieving patient-centered care. JAMA 2013;310(6):575–6.
37. Grunfeld E, Coule D, Whelan T, et al. Family caregiver burden: results of a longitudinal study of breast cancer patients and their principal caregivers. CMAJ 2004;170:1795–800.
38. Turan B, Goldstein MK, Garber AM, et al. Knowing loved ones' end-of-life health care wishes: attachment security predicts caregivers' accuracy. Health Psychol 2011;30(6):814–8.
39. Powazki R, Walsh D, Hauser K, et al. Communication in palliative medicine: a clinical review of family conferences. J Palliat Med 2014;17(10):1167–77.
40. Gueguen JA, Bylund CL, Brown RF. Conducting family meetings in palliative care: themes, techniques, and preliminary evaluation of a communication skills module. Palliat Support Care 2009;7(2):171–9.

41. Rhondali W, Dev R, Barbaret C, et al. Family conferences in palliative care: a survey of health care providers in France. J Pain Symptom Manage 2014;48: 1117–24.
42. Yennurajalingam S, Dev R, Lockey M, et al. Characteristics of family conferences in a palliative care unit at a comprehensive cancer center. J Palliat Med 2008;11: 1208.
43. Levin TT, Moreno B, Silvester W, et al. End-of-life communication in the intensive care unit. Gen Hosp Psychiatry 2010;32(4):433–42.

Spirituality in Geriatric Palliative Care

Christina M. Puchalski, MD, MS

KEYWORDS

- Spirituality • Palliative care • Geriatric • Empathic listening

KEY POINTS

- Patients value spiritual care.
- All clinicians should take a spiritual history; clinicians should engage patients about their spirituality, identify spiritual distress, and integrate patients' spirituality into holistic care plans.
- Validated tools exist to assess spirituality.
- Sincere, empathic listening can ease spiritual distress.

While covering for geriatrics and palliative care, I saw a new patient who had been in the intensive care unit for respiratory distress and was now transferred onto the medicine floor. I introduced myself and the resident with me, pulled up a chair, and proceeded to ask her about herself and what she understood was the reason she was in the hospital. I also asked her about her home life, what mattered most to her, what were her goals for her living, and I asked about her spirituality. She was delighted that two physicians actually sat down and listened to her and her whole story. "All these doctors and nurses come in and out and ask all these questions but never really listen to me—they are telling me how I should feel. Who am I to them? Just a number?"

People, regardless of age, want to be treated with respect, want to be really listened to, and want to be involved in their care. This is even more important in the geriatric population. As people age, they are challenged with more health issues, greater personal losses, and for many, an increased need to be dependent on others. Hearing or vision impairment or other medical conditions, such as cognitive impairment, can lead to difficulty in understanding. Respecting elderly patients means taking the time to be fully present and assuring them that we are listening to their whole story—not just the biomedical one.

Spiritual care is premised on the biopsychosocial spiritual model of care first described by Dame Cicely Saunders, the founder of the hospice and palliative care

George Washington Institute for Spirituality and Health, George Washington University School of Medicine, 2030 M Street NW Suite 4014, Washington, DC 20036, USA
E-mail address: cpuchals@gwu.edu

Clin Geriatr Med 31 (2015) 245–252
http://dx.doi.org/10.1016/j.cger.2015.01.011
0749-0690/15/$ – see front matter © 2015 Elsevier Inc. All rights reserved.

model.[1] Saunders further describes the concept of total pain, which refers to pain experiences, such as physical pain and/or psychosocial and spiritual suffering. Subsequent data has shown that physical pain can be exacerbated by psychosocial and spiritual distress so it is clinically important that total distress or pain be assessed adequately. This model, a whole-person model of care, describes all dimensions of a person as equally important in medical care and as a responsibility of all clinicians on the team.[2] There have many guidelines requiring spiritual care as an integral part of palliative care.[3,4] In a recent palliative care resolution passed by the World Health Organization, spiritual care was noted as a required part of palliative care.[5,6]

Spiritual care is care that honors the dignity of each patient served. It refers to deep listening as clinicians elicit the whole story of the patient, including what matters most to the patient and family. This care includes being compassionate and present to the suffering of the patient with a goal of attending to and alleviating all suffering and not just physical pain and other symptoms. To achieve that, it is important to do a spiritual screening or spiritual history to identify any spiritual distress and spiritual resources of strength of the patient and family and to integrate the patient's and family's spiritual beliefs, values, and practices into the care plan.

BACKGROUND

Research has demonstrated a relationship between spirituality and health outcomes, such as recovering from illness, improved health outcomes from surgery, finding meaning and will to live, and quality of life (QOL).[7–12] Spirituality and religion have also been shown to have an impact on how people cope with illness and suffering.[13–15] Spirituality has also been associated with an improved QOL for those with chronic and serious illness.[7] The literature supports the whole-person definition of QOL as encompassing the physical, psychological, social, and spiritual domains,[16–18] with spiritual well-being in one study found to be as significant as physical well-being.[19] A literature review found that half of the identified QOL instruments deemed appropriate for palliative care include items on spirituality, with most focusing on the existential aspects of spirituality related to meaning or purpose in life.[19] Spiritual well-being has been associated with lower levels of distress and a higher QOL across life expectancy prognoses.[20] Patients with cancer, for example, report feelings of anger and diminished self-esteem, which may be spirituality-related.[21] Conversely, patients with cancer also report their spirituality helped them find hope, gratitude, and positivity in their cancer experience,[8,22,23] and that their spirituality is a source of strength that helps them cope, find meaning in their lives, and make sense of the cancer experience as they recover from treatment.[24] One study found that 73% of patients with cancer expressed at least one spiritual need,[25] and that up to 40% of individuals with newly diagnosed and recurrent cancer showed a significant level of spiritual distress.[24]

Spirituality and health has grown during the last 30 years because of a resurgence in patients' interest in having more holistic and humanistic care. Although the origins of health care in the United States were primarily from religious organizations rooted in compassion and altruism, in the early 1900s, there was a split between the scientific and nonscientific aspects of care with spirituality and humanistic being relegated to the latter. It was not until the 1980s that interest in spirituality and health, in humanism, and in complementary and alternative medicine rose in part because of pressure from patients saying they want more holistic care.[26]

In the 1990s, medical schools began to develop courses on spirituality and health with spirituality being broadly defined. Initial efforts highlighted attention to patients' spirituality as a moral obligation of care that encouraged inclusion of spiritual care within medical education curriculum.[27] Increasing numbers of medical schools began to address the role of spirituality in their curricula in the last 20 years. More than 85% of US medical and osteopathic schools integrated topics related to spirituality into the curriculum.[28] This led to the development of competency behaviors in spirituality and health education[26] and triggered similar initiatives internationally. Now clinical guidelines for whole-person compassionate care, palliative care, and the biopsychosocial and spiritual model of care strongly recommend spiritual care for every patient.

In 2009, a national consensus conference, entitled Improving the Spiritual Domain of Palliative Care, developed a model of interprofessional spiritual care with recommendations of how to meet the spiritual needs of patients with serious and chronic conditions, thus applying this work to geriatrics and other patients.[2] The basic premise of this model is that all members of the clinical care team should address the spiritual needs of patients. The conference also defined spiritual distress as a diagnostic distress category based on the National Comprehensive Cancer Network distress guidelines.[29] The role of the interdisciplinary team was also discussed, with the chaplain as the spiritual care expert and the rest of the clinical team as the spiritual care generalists. It is not enough to simply refer to a chaplain; all clinicians need to engage patients and families about their spirituality and identify spiritual distress if present, formulate a diagnosis as part of the differential diagnosis of the patient's overall distress, and integrate the patient's spirituality into the care plan.

The consensus definition of spirituality is "spirituality is the aspect of humanity that refers to the way individuals seek and express meaning and purpose and the way they experience their connectedness to the moment, to self, to others, to nature, and to the significant or sacred."[2] The significant or sacred encompasses any expression of spirituality (religious, nonreligious, personal, philosophic, and so forth). Using these guidelines and findings, the National Comprehensive Cancer Network produced guidelines for the provision of interprofessional spiritual care. Clinicians should take a spiritual history. Other recommendations are as follows:

- All health care professionals should be trained in doing a spiritual screening or history as part of their routine history and evaluation.
- Spiritual screenings, histories, and assessments should be communicated and documented in patient records (eg, charts, computerized databases, and shared with the interprofessional health care team).
- Follow-up spiritual histories or assessments should be conducted for all patients whose medical, psychosocial, or spiritual condition changes, and as part of routine follow-up in a medical history.
- A spiritual issue becomes a diagnosis if the following criteria are met: (1) the spiritual issue leads to distress or suffering (eg, lack of meaning, conflicted religious beliefs, inability to forgive); (2) the spiritual issue is the cause of a psychological or physical diagnosis, such as depression, anxiety, or acute or chronic pain (eg, severe meaninglessness that leads to depression or suicidality, guilt that leads to chronic physical pain); and (3) the spiritual issue is a secondary cause or affects the presenting psychological or physical diagnosis (eg, hypertension is difficult to control because the patient refuses to take medications because of his or her religious beliefs).
- Treatment or care plans should include but not be limited to referral to chaplains, spiritual directors, pastoral counselors, and other spiritual care providers, including clergy or faith-community healers for spiritual counseling; development of spiritual goals; meaning-oriented therapy; mind-body interventions; rituals; spiritual practices; and contemplative interventions.

All members of an interdisciplinary team should respond to and address all dimensions of patient care: spiritual, religious, existential, physical, and psychological. Each of these components of care provides insight into the patient's suffering and his or her ability to manage that suffering. For this reason, spiritual discussions always should be a component of interdisciplinary team meetings. On the interdisciplinary team, each member has a specific role. In the inpatient setting the roles are as follows:

- The person doing the intake performs the initial screening. The goal of the screening is to identify patients in spiritual distress who need a chaplain referral urgently.
- The physician or nurse then takes the patient's spiritual history; in some settings, the social worker may take the spiritual history. The spiritual history is performed by those clinicians that develop treatment or care plans. The goal of the history is to identify spiritual issues that are resources of strength for the patient, or to identify a spiritual diagnosis or other spiritual issues that are affecting the patient's health or illness. In the interdisciplinary team, the chaplain can elaborate further on the clinician's initial assessment of the patient's spirituality.
- A spiritual assessment is a more detailed assessment of spiritual issues. The assessment is done by a board-certified or board-eligible chaplain. The previous model is a generalist-specialist model where the chaplain is the expert in spiritual care. Chaplains advise clinicians how to work with patients' spiritual issues and provide spiritual counseling as indicated. Chaplains also can coordinate the involvement of community spiritual care professionals, such as clergy, pastoral counselors, or spiritual directors. In addition, chaplains also may interact with faith community nurses, if patients' religious communities have these providers.
- The interdisciplinary team develops and implements the treatment or care plan; outcomes are measured with appropriate reevaluation and follow-up.

There are tools that can be used in the clinical setting for spiritual screening and history. Examples of such screening include one developed by Fitchett and Risk.[30] It is a two-question screening that includes "Are religion or spirituality important in your coping?" "How well are those working for you now?" A yes to the first question followed by a no to the second question indicates the need for a chaplain referral.

As the patient and family encounter the rest of the team, the clinicians would do a spiritual history as part of the social history and ask about spiritual distress as part of the review of systems for distress. Examples of spiritual histories include FICA,[31,32] SPIRIT,[33] (Spiritual belief system, Personal Spirituality, Integration, Rituals/restrictions, Implications, and Terminal events), and HOPE (Hope, Organized religion, Personal spirituality, Effects of care and decisions).[34] The FICA spiritual history has been validated with patients with cancer (**Table 1**).[35] Spiritual issues may also be apparent in the whole narrative of the patients' and families' stories (**Box 1**).

When these or other themes come up, clinicians can follow up with open-ended questions but listen specifically to the spiritual and psychosocial, cultural, or other context for these themes. Often letting a patient or family member have the attentive listening of a compassionate clinician as the patient or family member shares their issues helps the person resolve their issues. The clinician should recognize when a referral to a trained chaplain or a pastoral counselor or spiritual director might be helpful. Clinicians should always follow up with patients and families to see how they are dealing with their spiritual distress or other distress. In addition to identifying and diagnosing spiritual distress, the clinician should also identify spiritual resources of strength (**Box 2**).

Table 1 The FICA spiritual history tool	
FICA Tool	
F – Faith and Belief	Do you consider yourself spiritual or religious? or Do you have spiritual beliefs that help you cope with stress? If the patient responds "No," the physician might ask, "What gives your life meaning?" *Sometimes patients respond with answers such as family, career, or nature.*
I – Importance	What importance does your faith or belief have in our life? Have your beliefs influenced how you take care of yourself in this illness? What role do your beliefs play in regaining your health
C – Community	Are you part of a spiritual or religious community? Is this of support to you and how? Is there a group of people you really love or who are important to you? *Communities such as churches, temples, and mosques, or a group of like-minded friends can serve as strong support systems for some patients.*
A – Address in Care	How would you like me, your healthcare provider, to address these issues in your healthcare?

The FICA Spiritual History Tool is a validated tool for taking patients' spiritual history.
From Puchalski CM. The FICA spiritual history tool #274. J Palliat Med 2014;17(1):105–6; with permission.

THE WHOLE PERSON ASSESSMENT AND TREATMENT PLAN

Once spiritual issues are identified, they need to be addressed as part of the assessment and treatment plan. This plan should be based on the biopsychosocial and spiritual model of care, or what many have called "whole person care." An example of such a plan is presented next.

Brenda is an 86-year-woman admitted to the hospital for a right hip fracture. She had surgery to repair the hip fracture. She recently moved to this state to live closer

Box 1 Spiritual diagnosis
Existential distress
Lack of meaning or purpose
Anger at God or what people see as significant or sacred
Abandonment by God or what people see as significant or sacred
Conflicted belief systems
Despair
Hopelessness
Forgiveness or reconciliation needs
Specific religious or person ritual needs
Deep suffering and/or emptiness
Quest to deepen ones spiritual life

Box 2
Spiritual resources of strength

Spiritual beliefs, values, and practices that are supportive to the patient

Spiritual and religious support groups

Hope

Resiliency and good coping skills

Ability to find meaning and purpose

Having a supportive spiritual community

Experiencing connectedness to the moment, self, nature, or the significant or sacred

---

to her daughter and the daughter's family. On her spiritual history she reveals that her private belief in "something greater than ourselves" is very strong and has helped her get through many difficult times in her life including the death of her husband and youngest son in a plane crash many years ago. Family is what gives her most meaning so the loss is something she "will never get over." She expresses some regrets as she reviews her life and may need to look at some forgiveness issues, but overall is at peace. She is concerned that she will be a burden to her daughter, and this and her fear of not being as mobile as she was is causing some anxiety. She was affiliated with a spiritual community back home—she attends a Unitarian Church. She is now searching for a community here. She would also like to learn to meditate to help with her anxiety and would like to meet with someone to talk about her inner life as she is having some questions about life after death and the spiritual paths that she has taken in her life.

- Physical: postoperative pain management, discharge to skilled nursing facility for rehabilitation.
- Emotional: anxiety related to change in home, sense of burden with family, fear of losing some independence.
- Social: family meeting to discuss issues of being a burden and resources for increasing her independence.
- Spiritual: isolation from previous spiritual community, regret over issues in past with some desire for reconciliation, desire to explore her spiritual/inner life may be contributing to the anxiety. Referral to chaplain and spiritual director for a life review and further explorations of reconciliation, regret, and loss of previous state of functioning, which may be resulting in some meaning issues for her. She has spiritual strengths that help her be at peace. Her desire to meditate is positive as is searching for a new spiritual community.

This plan shows how important it is to address all dimensions of the patient's care. Spiritual suffering can significantly impact patient and family QOL and is therefore a critical aspect of good medical care delivery.

SUMMARY

The journey near the end of life is precious, difficult, and often tenuous. It is hard for patients and families to navigate this journey alone. Suffering includes psychosocial and spiritual distress. Often this suffering is profound and neglected. It is critical for clinicians to be fully present to the suffering to their patients and families. Deep presence is the key to spiritual care; listening to the inner story is essential. Tools help open the conversation, but it is who we are inherently—our presence, our commitment to serve and not abandon patients, and our desire to partner with patients—that makes a difference in our patients' and families' ability to cope with illness, stress, and loss.

REFERENCES

1. Saunders C. The treatment of intractable pain in terminal cancer. Proc R Soc Med 1963;56(3):195–7.
2. Puchalski C, Ferrell B, Virani R, et al. Improving the quality of spiritual care as a dimension of palliative care: the report of the consensus conference. J Palliat Med 2009;12(10):885–904.
3. American Academy of Hospice and Palliative Medicine, Center to Advance Palliative Care, Hospice and Palliative Nurses Association. National consensus project for quality palliative care: clinical practice guidelines for quality palliative care, executive summary. J Palliat Med 2004;7:611–27.
4. National Quality Forum. A national framework and preferred practices for palliative and hospice care: a consensus report. 2006. Available at: http://www.qualityforum.org/Publications/2006/12/A_National_Framework_and_Preferred_Practices_for_Palliative_and_Hospice_Care_Quality.aspx. Accessed January 21, 2015.
5. World Health Organization. Strengthening of palliative care as a component of integrated treatment within the continuum of care. 2014. Available at: http://apps.who.int/gb/ebwha/pdf_files/EB134/B134_R7-en.pdf. Accessed January 21, 2015.
6. Vitillo R, Puchalski C. World Health Organization authorities promote greater attention and action on palliative care. J Palliat Med 2014;17(9):988–9.
7. Cohen SR, Mount BM, Tomas JJ, et al. Existential well-being is an important determinant of quality of life: evidence from the McGill quality of life questionnaire. Cancer 1996;77(3):576–86.
8. Lynn Gall T, Cornblat MW. Breast cancer survivors give voice: a qualitative analysis of spiritual factors in long-term adjustment. Psychooncology 2002;11(6):524–35.
9. George LK, Larson DB, Koenig HG, et al. Spirituality and health: what we know, what we need to know. J Soc Clin Psychol 2000;19(1):102–16.
10. Jenkins RA, Pargament KI. Religion and spirituality as resources for coping with cancer. J Psychosoc Oncol 1995;13(1–2):51–74.
11. Koenig H, King D, Carson VB. Handbook of religion and health. New York: Oxford University Press; 2012.
12. Puchalski CM. Caregiver stress: the role of spirituality in the lives of family/friends and professional caregivers of cancer patients. Cancer caregiving in the United States. London: Springer; 2012. p. 201–28.
13. Vallurupalli MM, Lauderdale MK, Balboni MJ, et al. The role of spirituality and religious coping in the quality of life of patients with advanced cancer receiving palliative radiation therapy. J Support Oncol 2012;10(2):81.
14. Tarakeshwar N, Vanderwerker LC, Paulk E, et al. Religious coping is associated with the quality of life of patients with advanced cancer. J Palliat Med 2006;9(3):646–57.
15. Thune-Boyle IC, Stygall JA, Keshtgar MR, et al. Do religious/spiritual coping strategies affect illness adjustment in patients with cancer? A systematic review of the literature. Soc Sci Med 2006;63(1):151–64.
16. Ferrans CE. Development of a conceptual model of quality of life. Res Theory Nurs Pract 1996;10(3):293–304.

17. Ferrell BR, Grant M, Padilla G, et al. The experience of pain and perceptions of quality of life: validation of a conceptual model. Hosp J 1991;7(3):9–24.
18. Brady MJ, Peterman AH, Fitchett G, et al. A case for including spirituality in quality of life measurement in oncology. Psychooncology 1999;8(5):417–28.
19. Albers G, Echteld MA, de Vet HC, et al. Content and spiritual items of quality-of-life instruments appropriate for use in palliative care: a review. J Pain Symptom Manage 2010;40(2):290–300.
20. Adler NE, Page AE, editors. Cancer care for the whole patient: meeting psycho-social health needs. Washington, DC: National Academies Press; 2008.
21. Taylor EJ. Spiritual needs of patients with cancer and family caregivers. Cancer Nurs 2003;26(4):260–6.
22. National Cancer Institute. Facing forward: life after cancer treatment. 2014. Available at: http://www.cancer.gov/publications/patient-education/facing-forward. Accessed January 21, 2015.
23. Ferrell BR, Grant MM, Funk BM, et al. Quality of life in breast cancer survivors: implications for developing support services. Oncol Nurs Forum 1998;25(5): 887–95.
24. Astrow AB, Wexler A, Texeira K, et al. Is failure to meet spiritual needs associated with cancer patients' perceptions of quality of care and their satisfaction with care? J Clin Oncol 2007;25(36):5753–7.
25. Holland JC, Bultz BD. The NCCN guideline for distress management: a case for making distress the sixth vital sign. J Natl Compr Canc Netw 2007;5(1):3–7.
26. Puchalski CM, Blatt B, Kogan M, et al. Spirituality and health: the development of a field. Acad Med 2014;89(1):10–6.
27. Graves DL, Shue CK, Arnold L. The role of spirituality in patient care: incorporating spirituality training into medical school curriculum. Acad Med 2002;77(11):1167.
28. Association of American Medical Colleges: Report III. Contemporary issues in medicine. Medical School Objectives Project (MSOP III). 1999. Available at: http://academics.utep.edu/Portals/1887/Templates/time/contemporary_issues_in_med_commun_in_medicine_report_iii_.pdf. Accessed January 21, 2015.
29. National Comprehensive Cancer Network. Distress management. Clinical practice guidelines. J Natl Compr Canc Netw 2003;1(3):344.
30. Fitchett G, Risk JL. Screening for spiritual struggle. J Pastoral Care Counsel 2009; 63(1–2):4. Available at: http://journals.sfu.ca/jpcp/index.php/jpcp/article/view/71/57.
31. Puchalski CM. The FICA spiritual history tool #274. J Palliat Med 2014;17(1): 105–6.
32. Puchalski C, Romer AL. Taking a spiritual history allows clinicians to understand patients more fully. J Palliat Med 2000;3(1):129–37.
33. Maugans TA. The spiritual history. Arch Fam Med 1996;5(1):11–6.
34. Anandarajah G, Hight E. Spirituality and medical practice. Am Fam Physician 2001;63(1):81–8.
35. Borneman T, Ferrell B, Puchalski CM. Evaluation of the FICA tool for spiritual assessment. J Pain Symptom Manage 2010;40(2):163–73.

Public Health and Palliative Care in 2015

Mendwas D. Dzingina, MBBS, DLSHTM, MSc,
Irene J. Higginson, BM BS, BMedSci, PhD, FFPHM, FRCP, OBE, FMedSc*

KEYWORDS

- Public health • Palliative care • Cost-effectiveness • End-of-life
- Quality adjusted life year

KEY POINTS

- Palliative care is a public health concern, because the problems faced by patients and their families represent a substantial burden of illness and cost to society, which is likely to increase markedly in the future as the world's population continues to age.
- There is evidence to support palliative care services, but not yet enough information on the cost-effectiveness of many specific palliative care treatments/interventions.
- The lack of economic evaluations deprives decision makers of information required to best meet the needs of patients with progressive disease and at the end of life.
- It would be useful to empirically assess the appropriateness of generic measures of health-related quality of life (such as the EQ-5D) and the quality-adjusted life year framework in palliative care.

WHY IS PALLIATIVE CARE A MAJOR PUBLIC HEALTH CHALLENGE?
Palliative Care: Traditional Roots

The World Health Organization (WHO) defines palliative care as "an approach that improves the quality of life of patients and their families facing the problem associated with life-threatening illness, through the prevention and relief of suffering by means of early identification and impeccable assessment and treatment of pain and other problems, physical, psychosocial, and spiritual."[1,2]

The principles that underpin palliative care are based on the integration of symptom control, psychosocial care, and disease management, and so require true interdisciplinary collaboration. The goals of palliative care include improving patient and family quality of life,[3,4] satisfaction, and patients' perceptions of purpose and meaning of life.[5] Additionally, there is evidence to suggest that palliative care reduces emergency department attendances and hospital admissions toward the end of life and so provides benefits to the health care system and wider society.[6–8]

King's College London, Cicely Saunders Institute, Department of Palliative Care, Policy and Rehabilitation, Bessemer Road, London SE5 9PJ, UK
* Corresponding author.
E-mail address: irene.higginson@kcl.ac.uk

Clin Geriatr Med 31 (2015) 253–263
http://dx.doi.org/10.1016/j.cger.2015.01.002   geriatric.theclinics.com

Palliative care was initially developed in the British hospice movement in the 1960s. Guided by the pioneering work of Cicely Saunders, the concept evolved to include multidimensional needs of patients with a comprehensive approach practiced by a multidisciplinary team focusing initially, on end-of-life cancer patients attended to in hospices.

An early reference to palliative care being identified as a public health topic was published by Eric Wilkes[9] in the 1980s, following the recognition that most deaths were related to chronic conditions other than cancer, and that these occurred in hospitals and at home without any palliative care specialist intervention. On the basis of this reality, he proposed developing palliative care in all settings.

Global Health Policy

At the 67th World Health Assembly (May 23, 2014), the WHO passed the first ever resolution on palliative care recommending national health systems to provide palliative care in conjunction with potentially curative treatment, and not just as an optional extra.[6] The resolution also urges member states to develop and implement policies that support the integration of cost-effective and equitable palliative care services in the continuum of care, across all levels.[1]

Earlier resolutions regarding palliative care mainly focused on cancer patients and the end of life.[10] However, the WHO mandate on palliative care has evolved and currently extends to include patients with chronic noncancer conditions, in the early phase of their disease, as highlighted in the first ever palliative care resolution. It is evident that this evolution of the WHO mandate reflects the evolution of the concept of palliative care as a whole, which consists of

- Extending care beyond cancer and into more general chronic conditions
- Promoting early palliative interventions in the clinical evolution of the disease
- Applying palliative care measures in all settings of the health care system
- Identifying complexity versus prognosis as criteria for specialist interventions

In other words, the focus of palliative care has shifted from the concept of terminal illness to advanced chronic illness with a limited prognosis, and from a specialty (oncology) approach, to a national health care system approach.[10,11]

Aging Population and Shift in Causes of Morbidity and Mortality

According to the United Nations (UN), the life expectancy of the world's population has increased from 48 years from 1950 to 1955 to 68 years from 2005 to 2010.[12] This increase in life expectancy has been attributed to a decrease in mortality rates and a decline in fertility.[12] All regions of the world have experienced an increase in life expectancy, and this is predicted to increase in the future.[4,13,14] Currently, the pattern varies, with higher numbers of people dying in late old age in developed countries compared with lower and middle income countries. For example, Evans and colleagues[15] found that centenarian (a person aged 100 years or over) deaths increased by 56% between 2001 and 2010 in England.

The exact number of centenarians living worldwide is uncertain but is thought to be around 317,000 and is projected to rise to about 18 million by the end of this century.[15] In 2011, it was estimated that the 22% of the world's population was aged 60 years or older, and this proportion is expected to reach 32% in 2050 and 33% in 2100.[12] The number of persons aged 80 or over (oldest-old) is projected to increase almost eightfold in 2050.[4,12]

Over the last 6 decades, there has also been a shift in causes of morbidity and mortality. This shift can be attributed to 2 concepts of population transition: the demographic and epidemiologic theories of transition.[12,16] Demographic transition, characterized by a shift from high fertility and mortality rates to low fertility and mortality rates, leads to population aging (**Fig. 1**), which ultimately contributes to the change in patterns of causes of death witnessed in the last 6 decades.[16] This change in the predominant causes of death—away from a pattern dominated by communicable diseases toward one in which noncommunicable diseases (NCDs) account for the overwhelming majority of deaths—is referred to as epidemiologic transition.[12,16] Estimates from the UN show that in 2008, NCDs (eg, ischemic heart disease, cerebrovascular disease, chronic obstructive pulmonary disease, or lung cancer) accounted for 80% of deaths in developed countries, excluding Eastern Europe.[12]

In addition to this shift, there is greater comorbidity, with older people in the more advanced stages of illness often suffering several diseases, compounded with functional, sensory, or cognitive impairment.[4,17,18] Indeed the sickest 5% in health care, which includes mostly people with multiple comorbidities, may drive as much as half of health care spending,[19] thus suggesting that their needs should be addressed especially.

Current prevention and treatment efforts targeted at risk factors may delay or prevent the onset of NCD morbidity and mortality. Nevertheless, NCD morbidity and mortality are expected to increase as the world's population ages. This is primarily because the increase in NCD morbidity and mortality attributable to population aging is expected to greatly exceed the expected decline in NCD mortality attributable to preventative measures targeted at risk factors. In other words, although prevention strategies can reduce the burden of NCDs, the net burden is likely to be higher in the future because of population aging (**Table 1**).

Another issue related to population aging is the decrease in the proportion of younger people, and ratio of working-age to older people, as populations undergo epidemiologic transition.[20] This means fewer people, particularly women who have customarily been relied on to care for people at the end of life, will be able to find time to provide care for older people at the end of life. Moreover, because health systems vary in the degree to which they can provide resources to support home or institutional care for people at the end of life, some families will find the financial cost and burden of caring for older family members at the end of life unmanageable.[20]

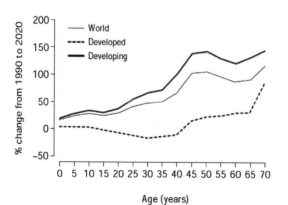

Fig. 1. Projected change in global population by age from 1990 to 2020. (*From* Murray CJ, Lopez AD. Alternative projections of mortality and disability by cause 1990–2020: Global Burden of Disease study. Lancet 1997;24:1503; with permission.)

Table 1
Leading projected causes of mortality for 2030 compared with 2015 causes

Disease	Predicted 2030 Ranking	Predicted 2015 Ranking
Ischemic heart disease	1	1
Stroke	2	2
Chronic obstructive pulmonary disease	3	4
Lower respiratory infections	4	3
Diabetes mellitus	5	8
Trachea, bronchus, lung cancers	6	7
Road injury	7	9
HIV/AIDS	8	6
Diarrheal diseases	9	5
Hypertensive heart disease	10	10

From WHO. Global health estimates summary tables: projection of deaths by cause, age and sex (xls:global summary projections). Available at: http://www.who.int/healthinfo/global_burden_disease/projections/en/. Accessed July 01, 2013; with permission.

Evidence of Unmet Palliative Care Need

According to WHO estimates, globally, about 20 million people (of whom 6% are children, and 67% are >60 years old) need palliative care annually.[2,21] This number doubles if those who could benefit from palliative care earlier in their illness are included.[2,6,21]

Cancer patients account for a third of people in need of palliative care. The rest include people suffering from a variety of chronic progressive diseases such as cardiovascular diseases, human immunodeficiency virus (HIV)/acquired immunodeficiency syndrome (AIDS), drug-resistant tuberculosis, chronic obstructive pulmonary disease, or renal failure.[6,21] The common causes of death among adults in need of palliative care are cardiovascular disease (38.5%), cancer (34%), chronic respiratory diseases (10.3%), and HIV/AIDS (5.7%).[2,21] It is conceivable that palliative care need will continue to increase as the world's population ages, so it is crucial to continue to measure palliative care need, using robust methods, to enable appropriate planning of services. Murtagh and colleagues[21] have recently developed a method for estimating palliative care need based on death registration data, incorporating both underlying and contributory causes of death. This method was found to be more appropriate for estimating palliative care need at a population level when compared with other pre-existing methods.[11,22,23]

INEQUITIES IN CARE
Poverty and Economic Deprivation

Evidence suggests that people in the lowest socioeconomic class tend to die younger, with poorer quality of life than those in higher socioeconomic classes.[24-26] Also, there are more hospital deaths in areas of high socioeconomic deprivation, despite preferences to the contrary.[25-27] Furthermore, because it tends to be more difficult to raise charitable funds for home and hospice care in deprived areas, the level of palliative care provision may be inversely proportional to the level of need—the inverse care law.[28] In addition to the complex range of factors that contribute toward the inverse care law, knowledge and awareness of palliative care and related services also appear to be important here. Koffman and colleagues[29] surveyed 252 cancer patients at 2 hospitals in London and found that the least materially deprived patients were significantly more likely to: recognize and describe the term palliative care (odds ratio [OR] = 8.4; P = .002) and understand the role of Macmillan nurses (OR = 6.68; P<.0001) when compared with their most deprived peers.

Older People

In many countries, older patients and their caregivers do not have equal access to palliative care when compared with younger patients.[30] This may partly be accounted for by the fact that most patients receiving palliative care are cancer patients, who on average, are younger; age, however, appears to be an independent factor both in place of death and access to specialist care. A systematic review by Burt and Raine[31] on the effect of age on referral to specialist palliative care reported that "older people were less likely to be referred to, or to use, specialist palliative care." Although this direct age discrimination is important, the main concern is perhaps that of indirect discrimination through failure to provide adequate palliative care to older people in the hospital. A European population-based survey by Gomes and colleagues[32] found that between 51% and 84% of people across 7 countries said they would prefer to die at home if they had advanced cancer. Despite this, 34% to 63% of deaths occurred in the hospital, and older people were found to be more likely to die in the hospital when compared with their younger counterparts.[33] Furthermore, a UK national end-of-life care survey of 473 bereaved informal care givers found that 75.6% of patients younger than 85 years were reported to have had an official record of preference for place of death, but this was only true for 39% of the oldest old (people aged 85 years and over).[34] The study also found that being over the age of 85 was associated with a 64% reduction in the odds of dying at home (OR = 0.36).[34]

Dementia

In recent years, dementia has become a major health challenge worldwide, and it accounts for increasing health resource use, particularly in higher income countries.[35] In 2005, the global prevalence of dementia was estimated to be 23.4 million, with an incidence of 4.6 cases annually (a new case every second).[36] The prevalence of dementia is expected to reach 81.1 million people by 2040, most of whom will live in lower income countries (60% in 2001, rising to 71% by 2040).[36] Research suggests that symptoms of dementia are similar to those of cancer; however, patients with dementia experience these symptoms for longer periods than those with cancer.[37] "Patients with dementia often receive poor end-of-life care, with inadequate pain control and without access to the palliative care services that patients with cancer are offered."[38]

Other Groups

Other disadvantaged groups include

- Black and minority ethnic groups
- People with learning disabilities
- Lesbian, gay, bisexual, and transgender groups
- Prisoners
- Refugees and asylum seekers
- Drug misusers
- Homeless people

PUBLIC HEALTH: OLD VERSUS NEW APPROACHES

Public health is concerned with the health of people at a population level.[39] It focuses on reducing morbidity and mortality and improving the health of communities, towns, cities, and nations. Because public health focuses on major causes of morbidity and mortality, it must evolve as the causes of morbidity and mortality change, as highlighted in the previous section. For example, while public health approaches in the 18th and 19th centuries focused on sanitary and environmental reforms,[40] and antibacterial therapies to curb transmission of communicable diseases (eg, cholera, tuberculosis, and malaria), which were the main causes of morbidity, the epidemiologic transition to NCDs in the 20th century necessitated the development of new public health approaches to addressing the problems posed by these killers of the new age.[16,41]

As a result, the new public health emerged with one of its main themes being that interventions be conducted with people rather than on people.[41] In essence, the main difference between the new and old public health is that the professional dominance of those from the outside — assuming that that they knew what was best for the community — was challenged.[41] For example, in the era of the old public health, health professionals adopted an institutionalized view toward hospice and end-of-life care (viewing death and dying as polluting experiences requiring containment, in hospice).[42] However, the ideas of the new public health and community empowerment promote moving away from the focus on containment of pollution and poverty to highlighting social and collective responsibility.[41]

The current public health approach to palliative care includes these ideas, and is an integral part of the wider global health promotion campaign. New initiatives are being developed that aim not only to promote the involvement of community members in care, but also in research. An example of such initiatives is the Patient, Family and Public Involvement (PPI)[43] in Palliative Care Research initiative, which is currently being developed at the Cicely Saunders Institute in London. The aims of the PPI initiative are primarily to: improve the quality, impact, and clinical relevance of palliative care research, and to demystify preconceptions and raise awareness of palliative care and palliative care research.[43]

EFFECTIVENESS AND COST-EFFECTIVENESS OF PALLIATIVE CARE

The effectiveness of palliative care can be considered at 2 levels. There is the general issue of the effectiveness of expert palliative care services and approaches, and there is also the effectiveness of individual new interventions, services, or approaches, including those that train those less experienced in palliative care.

There is now evidence to support expert (or specialist) palliative care multiprofessional teams. These appear to improve symptom control, reduce depression and psychological distress, in some instances improve patient quality of life, and in some studies improve survival.[7,8,44–48] They also can reduce care giver burden.[49] However, it should be stressed that these studies were carried out on services staffed usually by experts trained in palliative care. Therefore it is important that as palliative care services develop more widely outcomes are assessed on a routine basis, to ensure that the palliative care services continue to achieve high-quality outcomes for patients and families. Otherwise there may be a temptation for funders and commissioners of services to cut corners.[50,51]

There is, however, less evidence that specific training programs or pathways adapted from hospices and palliative care services and provided to generalists can improve care. The Liverpool care pathway failed to provide evidence of significant patient or care giver benefits in a cluster randomized controlled trial.[52] Many other training systems are in development but are not yet well evaluated. Equally, new techniques and treatments often need evaluation.

It is important for palliative care interventions to be routinely subjected to economic evaluation for at least 2 reasons. First, economic evaluation can enable comparisons between palliative care services to determine the most efficient use of currently allocated resources. "Services that can be shown to be relatively ineffective and costly can be replaced by those that achieve more for less."[53]

Second, and most importantly, palliative care will always compete with other health care services for the same funds. It is the responsibility of health policy makers to consider value for money when deciding what services to fund. Arguing for special consideration based on an intrinsic value of a service is rarely sufficient. Failure to demonstrate the cost-effectiveness of interventions can result in weak arguments in the competition for scarce resources.[53] Moreover, the WHO resolution on palliative care urges member states to develop and implement policies that support the integration of cost-effective and equitable palliative care services in the continuum of care, across all levels.[1] Therefore, to enable health policy makers to provide the resources required to meet the needs of dying patients, it is necessary for the palliative care community to provide information on the value for money of palliative care. Economic evaluation using cost-utility analysis, which compares interventions in terms of their cost per quality-adjusted life years (QALYs) gained, is a common means of providing such information.[54,55]

However, economic evaluations, particularly cost utility analyses of palliative care, are relatively rare, partly because of the difficulties of estimating costs and outcomes. For example, a 2014 review of the cost-effectiveness of palliative care found that: the majority of studies focused only on costs (cost analysis); only 1 study reported cost-effectiveness analysis, and none of the studies reported cost utility analysis.[56] The authors concluded that in most cases, palliative care was significantly cheaper than comparators.[56] "Economic evaluation of palliative interventions poses some challenges, both for palliative medicine and for economics."[53]

A major challenge around measuring cost in palliative care is that it is difficult to attribute true costs (and outcomes) to 1 particular service or intervention, because, within a single episode of illness, palliative care patients are usually cared for by various providers in different settings, simultaneously.[57] Also, because palliative care patients have complex needs and demands, it is necessary to adjust for need and complexity (case mix) when comparing costs between providers. It is reassuring that in several countries, palliative care funding models that account for case mix are being developed, such as: the Australian National Sub-acute and Non-acute Patient (AN-SNAP) system[58,59] and the current development work on a palliative-care currency in the United Kingdom.[60]

Although issues exist around measuring cost, the measurement of outcomes is arguably more challenging in the context of economic evaluations, particularly cost-utility analysis, of palliative care. This may partly be because some of the goals of palliative care, such as improving the quality of the experience of death, may be incompatible with how the QALY is estimated (ie, centered around maximizing healthy years or QALYs). There has been a lot of debate on the appropriateness of the QALY as an outcome measure in cost utility analyses of palliative care services.[53,61–65] A major criticism of the QALY framework is that standard tools, such as the EQ-5D[66,67] and SF-6D,[67] which have preference weights that enable the estimation of QALYs, are generic in nature, and so, do not capture specific domains that are important to palliative care.[62,64] Several validated palliative care-specific outcome measures exist, such as the Palliative Care Outcome Scale (POS),[68] and the McGill Quality of Life Questionnaire (MQOL),[69] which capture important palliative care domains. However, unlike the EQ-5D, these palliative care-specific outcome measures do not incorporate preference weights, and so cannot be used to estimate QALYs for cost utility analysis.

SUMMARY

Palliative care is a public health concern, because the problems faced by patients and their families represent a substantial burden of illness and cost to the society that is likely to increase markedly in the future as the world's population continues to age. There are also inequities in access to palliative care, continued unmet need. There is evidence to support palliative care services, but not yet enough information on the cost-effectiveness of many specific palliative care treatments/interventions. The lack of economic evaluations deprives decision makers of information required to best meet the needs of patients with progressive disease and at the end of life. These issues highlight the need for research in health economics and palliative care. It would be useful to empirically assess the appropriateness of generic measures of health-related quality of life (such as the EQ-5D) and the QALY framework in palliative care.

REFERENCES

1. WHO. Strengthening of palliative care as a component of integrated treatment within the continuum of care. 134th session: document EB134/28. 2014. Available at: http://apps.who.int/gb/e/e_eb134.html. Accessed September 01, 2014.
2. WHO. First ever global atlas identifies unmet need for palliative care. 2014. Available at: http://www.who.int/mediacentre/news/releases/2014/palliative-care-20140128/en/. Accessed September 01, 2014.
3. Hearn J, Higginson IJ. Outcome measures in palliative care for advanced cancer patients: a review. J Public Health Med 1997;19:193–9.
4. Hall S, Petkova H, Tsouros AD, et al. Palliative care for older people: better practices. Copenhagen (Denmark): World Health Organization; 2011.
5. Kaasa S, Loge JH. Quality of life in palliative care: principles and practice. Palliat Med 2003;17:11–20.
6. WHO. Sixty-Seventh World Health Assembly. Strengthening of palliative care as a component of integrated treatment throughout the life course (document A67/31). World Health Organization; 2014. Available at: http://apps.who.int/gb/e/e_wha67.html. Accessed September 01, 2014.
7. Gomes B, Calanzani N, Curiale V, et al. Effectiveness and cost-effectiveness of home palliative care services for adults with advanced illness and their caregivers. Cochrane Database Syst Rev 2013;(6):CD007760.
8. Higginson IJ, Evans CJ. What is the evidence that palliative care teams improve outcomes for cancer patients and their families? Cancer J 2010;16:423–35.
9. Wilkes E. Dying now. Lancet 1984;323:950–2.
10. Stjernswärd J, Colleau SM, Ventafridda V. The World Health Organization cancer pain and palliative care program past, present, and future. J Pain Symptom Manage 1996;12:65–72.
11. Gomez-Batiste X, Martinez-Munoz M, Blay C, et al. Identifying needs and improving palliative care of chronically ill patients: a community-oriented, population-based, public-health approach. Curr Opin Support Palliat Care 2012;6:371–8.

12. United Nations DoEaSA, Population Division (2012). Changing levels and trends in Mortality: the role of patterns of death by cause. United Nations publication, ST/ESA/SER.A/318, 2012. Available at: http://www.un.org/en/development/desa/population/publications/mortality/changingLevelsAndTrends.shtml. Accessed August 01, 2014.

13. Davies E, Higginson IJ. Better palliative care for older people. Copenhagen (Denmark): World Health Organizaton; 2004.

14. Davies E, Higginson IJ. Palliative care: the solid facts. Copenhagen (Denmark): World Health Organization; 2004.

15. Evans CJ, Ho Y, Daveson BA, et al. Place and cause of death in centenarians: a population-based observational study in England, 2001 to 2010. PLoS Med 2014; 11:e1001653.

16. Omran AR. The epidemiologic transition: a theory of the epidemiology of population change. Milbank Q 2005;83:731–57.

17. Kelley A, Meier D. Palliative care–a shifting paradigm. N Engl J Med 2010;363: 781–2.

18. Morrison RS, Meier DE. Geriatric palliative care. New York: Oxford University Press; 2003.

19. Meier DE. Focusing together on the needs of the sickest 5%, who drive half of all healthcare spending. J Am Geriatr Soc 2014;62:1970–2.

20. Davies E, Higginson IJ. Better Palliative Care for Older People. Copenhagen, Denmark: World Health Organization Europe; 2004. Available at: http://www.palliatief.nl/Service/Zoeken.aspx?q=publications. Accessed August 01, 2014.

21. Murtagh FE, Bausewein C, Verne J, et al. How many people need palliative care? A study developing and comparing methods for population-based estimates. Palliat Med 2014;28:49–58.

22. Higginson IJ. Palliative and terminal care. In: Stevens AR, Gabbay J, editors. Health care needs assessment. Oxford (England): Radcliffe Medical Press; 1997. p. 1–28.

23. Rosenwax LK, McNamara B, Blackmore AM, et al. Estimating the size of a potential palliative care population. Palliat Med 2005;19:556–62.

24. Gao W, Ho YK, Verne J, et al. Changing patterns in place of cancer death in England: a population-based study. PLoS Med 2013;10:e1001410.

25. Decker SL, Higginson IJ. A tale of two cities: factors affecting place of cancer death in London and New York. Eur J Public Health 2007;17:285–90.

26. Higginson IJ, Jarman B, Astin P, et al. Do social factors affect where patients die: an analysis of 10 years of cancer deaths in England. J Public Health Med 1999; 21:22–8.

27. Sims A, Radford J, Doran K, et al. Social class variation in place of cancer death. Palliat Med 1997;1:369–73.

28. Tudor Hart J. The inverse care law. Lancet 1971;297:405–12.

29. Koffman J, Burke G, Dias A, et al. Demographic factors and awareness of palliative care and related services. Palliat Med 2007;21:145–53.

30. Lock A, Higginson I. Patterns and predictors of place of cancer death for the oldest old. BMC Palliat Care 2005;4:6.

31. Burt J, Raine R. The effect of age on referral to and use of specialist palliative care services in adult cancer patients: a systematic review. Age Ageing 2006; 35:469–76.

32. Gomes B, Higginson IJ, Calanzani N, et al. Preferences for place of death if faced with advanced cancer: a population survey in England, Flanders, Germany, Italy, the Netherlands, Portugal and Spain. Ann Oncol 2012;23:2006–15.

33. Cohen J, Bilsen J, Addington-Hall J, et al. Population-based study of dying in hospital in six European countries. Palliat Med 2008;22:702–10.
34. Hunt KJ, Shlomo N, Addington-Hall J, et al. End-of-life care and preferences for place of death among the oldest old: results of a population-based survey using VOICES-Short Form. Palliat Med 2014;17:176–82.
35. Comas-Herrera A, Wittenberg R, Pickard L, et al. Cognitive impairment in older people: future demand for long-term care services and the associated costs. Int J Geriatr Psychiatry 2007;22:1037–45.
36. Ferri CP, Prince M, Brayne C, et al. Global prevalence of dementia: a Delphi consensus study. Lancet 2005;366:2112–7.
37. McCarthy M, Addington-Hall J, Altmann D. The experience of dying with dementia: a retrospective study. Int J Geriatr Psychiatry 1997;12:404–9.
38. Sampson EL, Ritchie CW, Lai R, et al. A systematic review of the scientific evidence for the efficacy of a palliative care approach in advanced dementia. Int Psychogeriatr 2005;17:31–40.
39. Institute of Medicine. The future of public health. Washinghton, DC: National Academy Press; 1998.
40. Szreter S. The importance of social intervention in Britain's mortality decline c.1850–1914: a re-interpretation of the role of public health. Soc Hist Med 1988;1:1–38.
41. Sallnow LK, Kumar S, Kellehear A. International perspectives on public health and palliative care. Milton Park; Oxfordhire (United Kingdom): Routledge; 2012.
42. Humphreys C. Tuberculosis, poverty and the first 'hospices' in Ireland. European Journal of Palliative Care 2003;10:164–7.
43. Daveson B, de Wolf-Linder S, Witt J, et al. Results of a transparent expert consultation on patient and public involvement in palliative care. Palliat Med 2014, in press.
44. Paiva CE, Faria CB, Nascimento MS, et al. Effectiveness of a palliative care outpatient programme in improving cancer-related symptoms among ambulatory Brazilian patients. Eur J Cancer Care (Engl) 2012;21:124–30.
45. Harding R, List S, Epiphaniou E, et al. How can informal caregivers in cancer and palliative care be supported? An updated systematic literature review of interventions and their effectiveness. Palliat Med 2012;26:7–22.
46. Gomez-Batiste X, Porta-Sales J, Espinosa-Rojas J, et al. Effectiveness of palliative care services in symptom control of patients with advanced terminal cancer: a Spanish, multicenter, prospective, quasi-experimental, pre-post study. J Pain Symptom Manage 2010;40:652–60.
47. Higginson IJ, Finlay IG, Goodwin DM, et al. Is there evidence that palliative care teams alter end-of-life experiences of patients and their caregivers? J Pain Symptom Manage 2003;25:150–68.
48. Finlay IG, Higginson IJ, Goodwin DM, et al. Palliative care in hospital, hospice, at home: results from a systematic review. Ann Oncol 2002;13(Suppl 4):257–64.
49. Higginson IJ, McCrone P, Hart SR, et al. Is short-term palliative care cost-effective in multiple sclerosis? A randomized phase II trial. J Pain Symptom Manage 2009;38:816–26.
50. Teno JM, Casarett D, Spence C, et al. It is "too late" or is it? Bereaved family member perceptions of hospice referral when their family member was on hospice for seven days or less. J Pain Symptom Manage 2012;43:732–8.
51. Teno JM, Gozalo PL, Lee IC, et al. Does hospice improve quality of care for persons dying from dementia? J Am Geriatr Soc 2011;59:1531–6.
52. Costantini M, Romoli V, Leo SD, et al. Liverpool care pathway for patients with cancer in hospital: a cluster randomised trial. Lancet 2014;383:226–37.

53. Normand C. Economics and evaluation of palliative care. Palliat Med 1996;10:3–4.
54. Earnshaw J, Lewis G. NICE guide to the methods of technology appraisal: pharmaceutical industry perspective. Pharmacoeconomics 2008;26:725–7.
55. Drummond MF, Sculpher MJ, Torrance GW, et al. Methods for the economic evaluation of health care programmes. 3rd edition. Oxford, UK: Oxford University Press; 2005.
56. Smith S, Brick A, O'Hara S, et al. Evidence on the cost and cost-effectiveness of palliative care: a literature review. Palliat Med 2014;28:130–50.
57. Murtagh FEM, Groeneveld EI, Kaloki YE, et al. Capturing activity, costs, and outcomes: The challenges to be overcome for successful economic evaluation in palliative care. Progress in Palliative Care 2013;21(4):232–5.
58. Gordon R, Eagar K, Currow D, et al. Current funding and financing issues in the Australian hospice and palliative care sector. J Pain Symptom Manage 2009;38:68–74.
59. Palmer KS, Agoritsas T, Martin D, et al. Activity-based funding of hospitals and its impact on mortality, readmission, discharge destination, severity of illness, and volume of care: a systematic review and meta-analysis. PLoS One 2014;9:e109975.
60. NHS-England. Developing a new approach to palliative care funding: A first draft for discussion. Leeds, UK; 2014. Available at: http://www.england.nhs.uk/2014/10/23/palliative-care/. Accessed August 01, 2014.
61. Gomes B, Harding R, Foley KM, et al. Optimal approaches to the health economics of palliative care: report of an international think tank. J Pain Symptom Manage 2009;38:4–10.
62. Normand C. Measuring outcomes in palliative care: limitations of QALYs and the road to PalYs. J Pain Symptom Manage 2009;38:27–31.
63. Round J. Is a QALY still a QALY at the end of life? J Health Econ 2012;31:521–7.
64. Hughes J. Palliative care and the QALY problem. Health Care Anal 2005;13:289–301.
65. Coast J, Smith RD, Lorgelly P. Welfarism, extra-welfarism and capability: the spread of ideas in health economics. Soc Sci Med 2008;67:1190–8.
66. Gusi N, Olivares PR, Rajendram R. The EQ-5D health-related quality of life questionnaire. In: Preedy V, Watson R, editors. Handbook of disease burdens and quality of life measures. New York: Springer; 2010. p. 87–99.
67. Marra CA, Woolcott JC, Kopec JA, et al. A comparison of generic, indirect utility measures (the HUI2, HUI3, SF-6D, and the EQ-5D) and disease-specific instruments (the RAQoL and the HAQ) in rheumatoid arthritis. Soc Sci Med 2005;60:1571–82.
68. Hearn J, Higginson IJ. Development and validation of a core outcome measure for palliative care: the palliative care outcome scale. Palliative Care Core Audit Project Advisory Group. Qual Health Care 1999;8:219–27.
69. Albers G, Echteld MA, de Vet HC, et al. Evaluation of quality-of-life measures for use in palliative care: a systematic review. Palliat Med 2010;24:17–37.

Palliative Care in the Era of Health Care Reform

Kavita Patel, MD, MS*, Domitilla Masi, MS

KEYWORDS

- Palliative care • Chronic disease • Health care reform
- Payment and delivery systems • Workforce challenges

KEY POINTS

- Patients with chronic diseases and advanced illnesses are an important population that could benefit from delivery system reforms, such as those in the Affordable Care Act.
- Research shows that palliative care achieves the health care reform goals of high-quality care and contained health care costs for patients with chronic and advanced illnesses.
- Several barriers restrict the uptake of palliative care; however, restructured payment mechanisms, educational and training systems, and messaging may increase access to these services.

BACKGROUND: OPPORTUNITIES FOR PALLIATIVE CARE

Patients with advanced illnesses or chronic care needs account for a disproportionate amount of US health care spending, yet research has shown that care for most of this population is average at best.[1] A recent Institute of Medicine report challenges the common notion that high health care expenditures are associated with the provision of care for patients in their last year of life, by highlighting that these "actively dying patients" constitute less than 13% of overall US health care spending.[2] In fact, most (90%) patients in the nation's top 5% highest-costing population, which account for 60% of total health care costs, are not in their last 12 months of life. Instead, a high proportion of this population (40%) is made up of patients with debilitating chronic or advanced illnesses, such as multiple sclerosis, Alzheimer disease and dementia, Parkinson disease, and schizophrenia, who have continual care needs but are not actively dying.[3] Although a significant share of US health care spending can be attributed to this population, patients and families often report low satisfaction with care; excessive burdens on caregivers; and inappropriately addressed symptoms

Engelberg Center for Health Care Reform, The Brookings Institution, 1775 Massachusetts Avenue, Northwest, Washington, DC 20036, USA
* Corresponding author.
E-mail address: KPatel@brookings.edu

Clin Geriatr Med 31 (2015) 265–270
http://dx.doi.org/10.1016/j.cger.2015.01.003
0749-0690/15/$ – see front matter © 2015 Elsevier Inc. All rights reserved.

and needs, exemplifying the provision of generally low-quality care.[4] Early access to palliative care, a specialized medical care that focuses on helping individuals with varying diagnoses and prognoses manage advanced illnesses, has been found to improve the quality of care for these patients.[5]

The alignment of delivery system reforms as a result of the Affordable Care Act and the goals of palliative care offer an important opportunity for action. New delivery models, such as accountable care organizations (ACOs), patient centered medical homes (PCMHs), and bundled/episodic payments focus on providing higher-quality and lower-cost care for complex patient populations. These goals are broadly achieved by paying groups of providers for the delivery of care that is better coordinated, delivered by a team, and focused on patient's needs. Similarly, palliative care is delivered through an interdisciplinary team of clinicians, chaplains, and social workers who collaborate to provide patients and families with high-quality care and support.[5] Studies show that palliative care decreases overall health care costs by lowering the provision of unnecessary services, hospital readmissions, emergency department use, and inpatient unit care, and by facilitating earlier referrals to hospice.[4] More importantly, these cost reductions occur through the provision of care that is better aligned with the goals of patients and their loved ones. For example, palliative care provides high-quality, patient-centered care by focusing on pain and symptom management, offering psychosocial support, and improving communication with patients and family members.[6]

However, although palliative care is recognized as a key service in achieving health care reform goals, the following section highlights how access to this care has been hindered by barriers relating to unstable payment structures, insufficient formal training, workforce shortages, and low provider and patient engagement. Policy proposals for greater uptake of these services include integrating palliative care into new payment and delivery models, reforming palliative care education and training, and improving messaging among providers and policy makers.

BARRIERS TO THE UPTAKE OF PALLIATIVE CARE

Palliative care is generally poorly reimbursed by public and private payers, which may discourage providers from taking up these services. Medicare, and some commercial insurers, only reimburse palliative care through their hospice benefit for patients who are at the end of life. The same applies for most state Medicaid benefit programs. This lack of reimbursement means that the cost of delivering early palliative care services, outside of hospice care, is absorbed by providers. Moreover, public and private payers only reimburse clinicians for the delivery of palliative care and do not pay for the services provided by other members of the interdisciplinary team, such as chaplains and social workers.[7] One payer that is actively trying to address this issue is Cambia Health Solutions, which insures more than 2.2 million people across 4 Northwestern states.[8] In the hope of creating a scalable model, Cambia has begun to pay providers for the delivery of palliative care, which includes reimbursement for the services of nonclinical staff, such as home health aides and social workers.[9]

A contributing factor to some of these barriers is that palliative care is a fairly new discipline. Although practiced informally before this time, palliative medicine officially became a subspecialty approved by the American Board of Medical Specialties in 2006.[10] Organizations such as the American Medical Association (AMA) and the American Association of Colleges of Nursing have tried to develop and promote palliative care training programs, yet standardized national curricula are still lacking for undergraduate and postgraduate education.[11] The closest effort in this arena is the Liaison Committee for Medical Education's mandate to incorporate end-of-life care training into all US medical schools.[12] Yet these educational programs are often heavily based on didactic courses, with limited practical clinical training components, and may perpetuate the misconception that palliative care is only provided at the end of life.

Barriers to formal training are often accompanied by workforce challenges. Although trends show that palliative care services have been increasing during the past decade, and that by 2014 84% of US hospitals with 50 or more beds will have palliative care services, today there are only approximately 5000 board certified palliative care specialists nationwide.[13,14] The American Academy of Hospice and Palliative Medicine predicts that only 4600 additional palliative care specialists will be produced within the next 20 years.[15] At the same time, estimates show a doubling of the population aged 65 years and older by 2030, suggesting that future demand for this specialty will outstrip supply.[16] Beyond physicians specialized in palliative care, other clinicians who care for patients with advanced illnesses also have limited palliative care expertise.[4] For example, only a small percentage of family physicians gain additional training, including in areas such geriatrics and palliative care.[17] Further, the shortage of palliative care providers is even more severe in rural areas, where the need for such care is in greater demand given a higher percentage of more ill, low-income, and elderly patients.[18]

Finally, low provider acceptance and patient awareness/engagement, because of common misconceptions about palliative care, are major barriers to referral and access. Palliative care relies on referrals from other providers; however, a survey of specialist physicians providing care to patients with lung cancer in New York City found that almost half (48%) of the 155 respondents referred less than 25% of their patients to palliative care consultations.[19] Many physicians erroneously believe that palliative care services are only provided with hospice and end-of-life services, and cannot be provided alongside life-prolonging therapies. In fact, studies find that providers often refer patients to palliative care services based on their prognosis, and referrals are typically made at points of crisis, late in the disease course, and close to the end of life.[20–22] Similar misconceptions about palliative care held by the public may also incite fear among providers that referrals to palliative care will be perceived as "giving up" by their patients.[21] Public opinion research found that in 2011, 70% of Americans had no knowledge of palliative care.[23] Lack of patient familiarity with palliative care may inhibit access to services through hindering patients from seeking this care from their providers.

EXPANDING ACCESS TO PALLIATIVE CARE: POLICY RECOMMENDATIONS AND PROPOSALS

Palliative care should be integrated into new models of payment and delivery, such as PCMHs and ACOs, to tackle unstable payment structures and increase access to these services. Private payers have been leading these initiatives. For example, the ACO formed by Anthem Blue Cross and HealthCare Partners in California, which recently announced creating $4.7 million in savings within 6 months, included the provision of palliative care services for its high-risk patient population.[24] The Department of Family Medicine PCMH at the University of California Los Angeles, which focuses on patients with complex, debilitating physical and mental illnesses, has structurally embedded a specialized pain management and palliative care clinic in its center.[25] Preliminary data show that access to the clinic has created high levels of patient and family member satisfaction, along with decreases in hospital admissions and emergency department visits for patients.

Business models such as Aspire Health, partly funded by BlueCross BlueShield Venture Partners, facilitate the integration of palliative care services into new delivery models. Aspire Health is a home- and outpatient-based palliative care provider that creates independent physician practices that partner with ACOs and other new delivery systems.[22] Practices are run by interdisciplinary care teams consisting of specialized physicians and nurse practitioners, who are available to patients on a 24/7 basis, and social workers, nurses, and chaplains, depending on a specific patient's needs.[26] Aspire Health has developed and implemented sophisticated algorithms that allow practices to identify patients who are in need of palliative care services, and an electronic health record (EHR) system that focuses specifically on palliative care treatment and facilitates data-sharing with a patient's primary care practitioner (PCP). Results from Aspire Health's pilot indicate a significant decrease in hospitalizations and 70% of patients being discharged to hospice, with a doubling in the median length of stay once in hospice.[22] Experts have suggested that the implementation of automated referral triggers in EHRs lightens workflow burdens for physicians and increases referrals by up to 50%.[27] However, for these models to become scalable, the development of standardized quality metrics specific to palliative care is necessary.

Palliative care workforce shortages can be overcome by reforming palliative care education and training. Payment and delivery system transformation alone will not increase the uptake of palliative care services if scarcities in specialized physicians persist. Common recommendations include lifting the current general medical education cap on palliative care training, enhancing funding for fellowship programs, and implementing standardized curricula for undergraduate and postgraduate training.[28,29] However, another way of mitigating current and future palliative care specialist shortages is to improve access to palliative care training among all physicians caring for patients with debilitating chronic or advanced illnesses, including those in specialties such as general internal medicine, cardiology, hematology/oncology, pulmonary/critical care, and neurology, among several others. A suggested coordinated model is one in which patients' basic palliative care needs, such as simple pain and symptom management and goals of treatment discussions, are fulfilled by treating physicians, who only refer the more complex patients to palliative care specialists.[14]

Palliative care education can also be proliferated through partnerships between professional societies and academic institutions. For example, a Project to Educate Physicians on End-of-life Care developed by Institute for Ethics at the AMA, which includes palliative care training, has been circulated to more than 90,000 practicing physicians nationwide.[29] Internet-based education can also be effectively used as a low-cost way of providing palliative care training, especially in light of limited numbers of educators specialized in palliative care and diminished access to training in rural areas. For example, the Extension for Community Healthcare Outcomes (ECHO) program, created by the University of New Mexico, uses video conferencing technology to train PCPs in palliative care. Results have shown that outcomes of palliative care provided by the ECHO program are equitable to those delivered in academic settings. This model is now being used nationally and internationally.[30]

Finally, although payment and education system reforms are key in ultimately increasing access to palliative care, their uptake depends highly on improving communication strategies when explaining the services to various stakeholders. Teaching providers the use of appropriate introductory language is essential for increasing referrals to palliative care. Ninety percent of Americans are found to be "very or somewhat likely" to contemplate palliative care for family members with an advanced illness after receiving an appropriate explanation of the services.[5] Another study found that altering the name from *palliative* to *supportive* care accelerated referrals to these services.[11] From a policy standpoint, to prevent "death panel" discussions, as was the case during 2009 deliberations over simply reimbursing for a service to better understand patients' preferences at the end of life, policy debates must highlight palliative care's goals of improving patient quality of life while not diminishing survival.[28]

REFERENCES

1. Meier DE. Increased access to palliative care and hospice services: opportunities to improve value in health care. Milibank Q 2011;89(3):343–80.
2. Institute of Medicine. Dying in America: improving quality and honoring individual preferences near the end of life. Washington, DC: The National Academies Press; 2014. Available at: http://books.nap.edu/openbook.php?record_id=18748. Accessed October 10, 2014.
3. Meier DE. IOM report calls for transformation of care for the seriously ill. Health Affairs Blog; 2014. Available at: http://healthaffairs.org/blog/2014/09/24/iom-report-calls-for-transformation-of-care-for-the-seriously-ill/. Accessed January 12, 2015.
4. Meier DE. Improving health care value through increased access to palliative care. NIHCM Foundation; 2012. Available at: http://www.nihcm.org/images/stories/NIHCM-EV-Meier_FINAL.pdf.
5. Lindvall C, Hultman TD, Jackson VA. Overcoming the barriers to palliative care referral for patients with advanced heart failure. J Am Heart Assoc 2014;3(1): e000742.
6. Fletcher DS, Panke JT. Opportunities and challenges for palliative care professionals in the age of health reform. J Hosp Palliat Nurs 2012;14(7):452–9.
7. Lubell J. Easing their pain: palliative care grows despite reimbursement issues. Modern Healthcare 2010;40:30, 32–3. Available at: http://www.modernhealthcare.com/article/20100531/MAGAZINE/100529913.
8. The Daily Briefing. Why one insurer is launching a major palliative care program. The Advisory Board Company; 2014. Available at: http://www.advisory.com/daily-briefing/2014/06/19/why-one-insurer-is-launching-a-major-palliative-care-program. Accessed October 9, 2014.
9. Evans M. Insurer begins huge palliative care program. Kaiser Health News 2014. Available at: http://kaiserhealthnews.org/news/insurer-begins-huge-palliative-care-program/.
10. Physician Certification. Physician board certification in hospice and palliative medicine (HPM). National Hospice and Palliative Care Organization; 2006. Available at: http://www.nhpco.org/palliative-care/physician-certification. Accessed October 8, 2014.
11. Von Gunten C, Ferrell B. Palliative care: a new direction for education and training. Health Affairs Blog; 2014. Available at: http://healthaffairs.org/blog/2014/05/28/palliative-care-a-new-direction-for-education-and-training/.
12. Horowitz R, Gramling R, Quill T. Palliative care education in us medical schools. Med Educ 2014;48(1):59–66.
13. Center to Advance Palliative Care. Growth of palliative care in U.S. hospitals 2013 snapshot. Available at: https://www.capc.org/media/filer_public/0d/db/0ddbecbc-8dc7-449d-aa50-584960f18880/capc-growth-analysis-snapshot-2013.pdf. Accessed October 8, 2014.

14. Quill TE, Abernethy AP. Generalist plus specialist palliative care – creating a more sustainable model. N Engl J Med 2013;368:1173–5.
15. Forum news & updates. Palliative care in need of more doctors. American Hospital Association Web site. Available at: http://www.ahaphysicianforum.org/news/enews/2012/091312.html#08. Accessed October 9, 2014.
16. Shih YT, Hurria A. Preparing for an epidemic: cancer care in an aging population. ASCO University; 2014. Available at: http://meetinglibrary.asco.org/content/114000133-144. Accessed October 14, 2014.
17. American Academy of Family Physicians. Aligning resources, increasing accountability, and delivering a primary care physician workforce for America. Available at: http://www.aafp.org/dam/AAFP/documents/advocacy/workforce/gme/FullGME-090914.pdf. Accessed October 14, 2014.
18. Rural palliative care. StratisHealth. Available at: http://www.stratishealth.org/expertise/longterm/palliative.html. Accessed October 14, 2014.
19. Smith CB, Nelson JE, Berman AR, et al. Lung cancer physicians' referral practices for palliative care consultation. Ann Oncol 2012;23(2):382–7.
20. Kavalieratos D, Mitchell EM, Carey TS, et al. "Not the 'grim reaper service':" an assessment of provider knowledge, attitudes, and perceptions regarding palliative care referral barriers in heart failure. J Am Heart Assoc 2014;3:e000544.
21. Schenker Y, Crowley-Matoka M, Dohan D, et al. Oncologist factors that influence referrals to subspecialty palliative care clinics. J Oncol Pract 2014;10(2):e37–44.
22. Smith B, Lasher A. Aspire health's approach to palliative care [webinar]. NIHCM Foundation; 2014. Available at: http://www.nihcm.org/improving-access-to-integrated-palliative-care. Accessed October 6, 2014.
23. Center to Advance Palliative Care. 2011 public opinion research on palliative care: a report based on research by public opinion strategies. Available at: https://www.capc.org/media/filer_public/18/ab/18ab708c-f835-4380-921d-fbf729702e36/2011-public-opinion-research-on-palliative-care.pdf. Accessed October 6, 2014.
24. HealthCare Partners. Anthem Blue Cross and HealthCare Partners saves $4.7 million in six months [press release]. Available at: http://www.healthcarepartners.com/NewsRoom/releasedetails.aspx?rid=53. Accessed October 7, 2014.
25. Wallensetein DJ. Palliative care in the patient-centered medical home. Prim Care 2012;39(4):627–31.
26. BusinessWire. Frist's Aspire Health announces expansion into four new states; receives funding from BlueCross BlueShield Venture Partners. Available at: http://www.businesswire.com/news/home/20140624006539/en/CORRECTING-REPLACING-Frist%E2%80%99s-Aspire-Health-Announces-Expansion#.VEaltT_In08. Accessed October 7, 2014.
27. The Advisory Board Company. Five characteristics of programs that capture the full value of palliative care. Available at: http://www.advisory.com/~/media/Advisory-com/Research/PEC/Resources/Posters/Palliative-Care/28097_PEC_Palliative_Care_Poster.pdf. Accessed October 10, 2014.
28. Parkin RB, Kirch RA, Smith TJ, et al. Early specialty palliative care—translating data in oncology into practice. N Engl J Med 2013;369(24):2347–51.
29. Von Roenn JH, Voltz R, Serrie A. Barriers and approaches to the successful integration of palliative care and oncology practice. J Natl Compr Canc Netw 2013;11:S11–6.
30. Marr L, Neale D. Project ECHO: bringing palliative care consultation to rural New Mexico through a novel telemedicine format. J Pain Symptom Manage 2012; 43(2):448–9.

Culturally Relevant Palliative Care

 CrossMark

Richard Payne, MD[a,b,*]

KEYWORDS

• Culture • Palliative care • Imagination • Narrative competency

KEY POINTS

- Although all persons facing serious illness have individual needs, the foundation for providing quality palliative care is in making connections that focus on universal human needs.
- Clinicians should make considered and reflective judgments that minimize stereotyping and superficial generalizations.
- Clinicians should be open to the perspective of the person experiencing illness and suffering.
- The story of illness should be encouraged and elicited for a fuller, richer perspective of the person with illness who is like all others, like some others, and like no others.

"Every person is like all others, like some other, and like no others."
    —Adopted from Kluckhohn and Murray, 1948

ONE PERSON—3 IDENTITIES

This proverb or witticism[1,2] is relevant for all clinicians. Proverbs or writings of this kind can be considered part of a larger genre of "wisdom literature."[3] Perhaps the most famous examples of wisdom literature are the Old Testament books of Job, Psalms, Ecclesiastes, and, of course, the book of Proverbs. By using techniques such as simile, symbolism and allegory—language that likens one thing to another, and makes comparisons to understand the relative values of concepts—these phrases, scripture passages, and secular witticisms provide concentrated nuggets of wisdom to assist with navigating a world that is not black and white, but full of shades of gray.

This particular expression points to a great challenge for clinicians who desire to practice competent, comprehensive care, attentive to the particular human needs of

[a] The Divinity School, Duke University, Box 90968, Durham, NC 27708-0968, USA; [b] Bioethics, Center for Practical Bioethics, Kansas City, MO 64105, USA
* Corresponding author. The Divinity School, Duke University, Box 90968, Durham, NC 27708-0968.
E-mail address: rpayne@div.duke.edu

Clin Geriatr Med 31 (2015) 271–279
http://dx.doi.org/10.1016/j.cger.2015.01.010
0749-0690/15/$ – see front matter

their patients. Analogous to the 3 physical states of water, which can exist as a solid, a liquid, or a gas, and still be constituted of the same fundamental substances—2 hydrogen atoms and 1 oxygen atom—persons experiencing illness exist in 3 interrelated states or identities. Attention to the multiplicity of perspectives of individuals rendered vulnerable by illness is at the heart of providing competent and humane medical care. Recognizing that every person is "like all others" identifies the notion of a shared common humanity and universal needs when facing serious and life-limiting illness. Recognizing that every person is "like some others" acknowledges that we share commonalities with certain tribal and cultural groups and not with others. Finally, affirming that every person is "like no others" speaks to the very important need to individualize care and to assess the specific circumstances of illness and the particular needs of individuals with unique preferences and personal values.

Like All Others

It has been said that "our confrontation with death lays bare the spiritual dimension of the human experience" (Ira Byock, personal communication, 2004). This idea speaks to a nearly universal yearning for understanding of the connection to other peoples, to wonder about creation, and perhaps a Creator, and to find meaning and purpose in life experiences—in the context of serious illness and contemplating a life that is perhaps about to end. The imminent loss of self, or loss of a loved one, often directs one to important spiritual values that transcend racial, gender, class, and geographic boundaries. These spiritual values may be enriched by and interpreted through specific religious traditions and rituals. These values—the desire not to be alone or abandoned during illness, but to be in the company of family and loved ones; the desire to be free of physical pain and avoidable suffering; the desire to reconcile with and say goodbye to family and loved ones—undergird nearly universal human aspirations in the context of serious illness and end-of-life care. These values transcend the common social and political categorizations of human life. Professional caregivers can make valid assumptions that these values and needs will apply to all of those they serve—irrespective of race, ethnicity, religious tradition, and socioeconomic status.

Like Some Others

Although these values and aspirations are shared by the human family, the ways in which these needs and desires are voiced, the meanings attached to these values, and the way people act on them are influenced greatly by the nuances and characteristics that make up the rich diversity of the human species. The great common ground of human concerns that make everyone "like all others" is often confounded in the distinctive cultures of community and the personality that defines ethnic groups and individuals. In this context, everyone is "like some others" in the common cultural patterns that bind people together in community. But even here, there are important caveats. Culture and community often refers to groups of individuals who share a common language, lifestyle, and worldview.[4] Community may be geographically defined or virtual, unencumbered by physical limitations of space and time. Adding to the complexity, notions of community and culture may overlap and cross boundaries between racial and ethnic categories making conventional categorizations problematic and not at all predictive of the ways in which people are likely to response to serious illness, disease, and loss. In fact, even in the expression and discussion of firmly held medical "facts," clinicians must be sensitive to notions of cultural interpretation. Perhaps the best example of this is the recent controversies concerning the acceptance of "brain death" as the legal and practical criteria for actual death (see VALUES AND CULTURAL PERSPECTIVES DETERMINE THE "RIGHT ANSWER").

Like No Others

To say that humans are all individuals is a simple truism. The universality of human spiritual concerns noted are uniquely modified and influenced by individual prefer- ences, practices, and values—in the case of spirituality, by the particularities of religious perspectives. In fact, many theologians, faith leaders, and even secular phi- losophers–bioethicists often reject the legitimacy and ultimately the usefulness of "generic" kinds of spiritual understanding of the world that do not account for the cus- toms and teachings embodied in a specific (religious) tradition.[5] Daniel Callahan, a prominent and highly influential bioethicist, although admitting the decline of impor- tance of religion in his personal life, has nonetheless advocated for greater voice by theologians and religious thinkers in the bioethics dialogue because the lack of reli- gious perspectives:

> "First of all, [makes us] to heavily dependent upon the law as the working source of morality... It leaves us, secondly, bereft of the accumulated wisdom and knowl- edge that are the fruit of long-established religious traditions... It leaves us, thirdly, forced to pretend that we are not creatures both of particular moral communities and the more sprawling, inchoate general community that we celebrate as an expression of our pluralism."[6]

Clinicians who wish to practice "holistically," respectful of the 3 coexistent identities of persons who are experiencing illness, must witness and appreciate an individuality that is built on a foundation of common humanity, but nonetheless are also critically influenced by "particular moral communities," in the words of Callahan. The distinctive- ness of culture, language, social circumstance, religion, personality, and gender are key foundations by which individuals find meaning and purpose in their living and dying and come to terms with the loss and remembrance of family and loved ones. In the final analysis—and paradoxically—one must tap into the commonalities of humanity and at the same time have the desire and skill to learn about and to come to understand the particularities of the person. Only then can palliative care clinicians truly engage with patients and families to find meaning in illness, death, and loss.

VALUES AND CULTURAL PERSPECTIVES DETERMINE THE "RIGHT ANSWER"— INTERPRETING BIOETHICS AND MEDICAL DECISION MAKING IN THE REAL WORLD

A renowned bioethicist and health policy expert recently gave a lecture, and during the discussion of a controversial health policy topic relating to the extent to which access to health care services should be limited to individuals, the author asked to what extent the "answers," in terms of health policy solutions, depend on perceptions of po- litical power dynamics and concerns about transparency (or the lack thereof) of the motives of policymakers. The response (paraphrased) was, "I don't worry about the power dynamics, I just want to get the 'right' solution."

However, other bioethicists, such as Bruce Jennings, assert that even in the realm of ethics—reasoning about what ought to be done—no one can escape the powerful influence of cultural perspectives.

The advance of human capacity to manipulate the conditions of life is generally referred to as "biotechnology," and the extension of the domain of human agency that it brings about may be referred to as "biopower." Whenever there is an innovative, substantial, and rapid extension of human power—as is happening now frequently, but never really routinely with biotechnology—society must come to grips not only with the scientific and political implications of that power but also with its cultural meaning.[7]

All individuals perceive and define important ethical and moral concepts such as autonomy, justice, beneficence, and nonmalfeasance through a filter of their general understanding of the world, their place in a "particular moral community," and their specific life experiences. A good example of the tensions that occur when there is a dissonance between medical expert pronouncements of the "right medical answer" and cultural norms and acceptance of these judgments by patients and families can be found in the recent controversies concerning brain death determinations.

Recall that the current conceptualization of brain death originated with the seminal publication of the Harvard Medical School Committee on the Determination of Brain Death,[8] and the endorsement of these recommendations by the President's Commission on Bioethics[9] several years later, and reaffirmed in 2008 (albeit with minority dissent within the commission).[10] These publications established that the irreversible damage of the brain—cortex and brainstem—was essential "death," and this definition has become the legally accepted standard of death in all 50 states since 1970. However, as evidenced by recent high-profile media cases, there is significant resistance to this seemingly "settled" medical consensus, particularly among racial ethnic and religious minority groups.

Consider the case of Jahi McMath, the adolescent African-American girl declared brain dead after surgical complications of a tonsillectomy. Her parents did not accept this diagnosis, insisting that she is not "dead" on the basis of their observations of her, and also alleging that the hospital's motives for determining brain death was to avoid medical expenses associated with her care and possibly to minimize medical liability. Her parents eventually petitioned transfer to a long-term care facility in New Jersey, one of two states that permit religious exceptions to the declaration of brain death.

Of note, the patient is still being "maintained" on artificial means of life support now approximately 1 year after the determination of "brain death" (albeit with no firm evidence of a return to any semblance of consciousness; she remains completely dependent for all aspects of care). However, assuming that the initial declaration of brain death was correct and done in accordance with rigorous medical criteria, the fact that she has not experienced circulatory failure 1 year after being declared "dead" challenges basic cultural and religious teachings and tradition about when death occurs, and even challenges basic common sense assumptions of everyday experience about death and dying. It is no accident that this and other cases challenging the notion of whole brain death as "death" are being brought forth by members of ethnic and racial minority communities and individuals with strong religious convictions on the moral correctness of this approach, because these groups are not represented usually by those with power and authority in the medical establishment. In a sense, it should come as no surprise that the notion of whole brain death as being the legal basis for death is being attacked as an illegitimate concept in a society in which there is a diversity of experience and cultural teachings about death and dying, even though there is still nearly universal medical acceptance that brain death is equivalent to biological death. So, getting the "right" answer to important medical and health policy questions such as, "Is death of the whole brain necessary and sufficient to death of person in legal and social terms?" requires both a combination of medical expertise and an understanding of individuals' diverse beliefs. Some individuals define death—and the essence of being human—in different terms that others who take a singularly focused biological view. **Box 1** lists some of the social and cultural determinants of resistance to expert medical and bioethics consensus on controversial problems such as brain death.

However, respect for diversity and individual preferences raise questions that go beyond the considerable challenges of being aware and tolerant of different views.

Box 1
Social and political determinants of perceptions of health policies (such as "brain death")

- Ability to connect to others with similar perspectives—facilitated by the advent of the Internet

- Erosion of trust in the integrity of institutions and the professions—facilitated by political, ethical, and financial scandals

- Potential impact of contemporary health care practices—facilitated by:
  - Health care funding crises
  - Medical malpractice debates
  - State-by-state tinkering with concepts of life and death

Adapted from Greenberg G. Lights out: a new reckoning for brain death. The New Yorker, Jan 15, 2014.

To what extent should clinicians attempt to meet the individualized needs, preferences, and requests of the sick individual? Are all individual preferences, intentions, and motivations legitimate? What about the individual who only feels "comfortable" with another individual or member of their community because they are acting on racist emotions about the inferiority or differences of another group? What about the legal obligations of individuals and institutions to uphold nondiscrimination laws? The courts have ruled that there are limits to the degree to which an individual's racial preferences may be accommodated in health care settings.[11] Questions such as these raise important challenges to notions of the primacy of personal autonomy and the appropriateness, or even legality, of responding to all individual preferences. The best strategy for clinicians who wish to act in good faith toward controversial requests for personalized care is to always proceed with a motivation to do what is ethical, legal, and appropriate to facilitate meaning-making and "healing" for that person.

GREAT PALLIATIVE CARE CLINICIANS ARE TECHNICALLY COMPETENT AND FULLY PRESENT—AND THEY HAVE IMAGINATIONS

These caveats notwithstanding, how does the palliative care clinician come to terms with the complexities of the "3-identity individual" so that comprehensive assessments and treatment recommendations truly address the essence of their needs, in all dimensions of experience and expectation?

First and foremost, clinicians and patients should relate to each other across a common humanity. This may require the clinician, especially the physician, to unburden himself or herself from the "white coat mentality" when this interferes with sharing and communication, and when it reinforces notions of power and privilege that compromise the ability to "see" suffering.

It is crucial for palliative care clinicians to open their imaginations to "see" the world as their patients may be seeing the world. This offers a remarkable opportunity to gain insight into the patients' sources of distress and suffering, and allows for perspectives on how clinicians can more effectively attend to this suffering. This opening of the imagination is facilitated by embracing the commonalities of human experience and human nature shared by clinician and patient.

Evidence-based medicine directs critical core competencies of clinicians to practice their professions in highly skillful and effective ways. Randomized controlled trials, comparative effectiveness studies, and other forms of empirical clinical research that form the basis for establishing "evidence" for best medical practice take advantage of important broad commonalities among diverse individuals and populations so that important generalizations can be made. This evidence provides the basis for standardizing care and defining quality metrics. Highly effective clinicians, who provide "good doctoring and nursing" are critically dependent on having the knowledge and expertise that flows from population-based medical research.

At the same time, great clinicians are also called to practice "culturally competent" care, or care that assesses sick persons and makes treatment recommendations based on a sense of the cultural and personal values of individuals. To do this effectively requires a fundamental increased self-awareness and receptivity on the part of clinicians to the connections between "worldview, beliefs, norms and behaviors related to health, illness and care-seeking in different populations."[12] Clinicians should be aware of and acknowledge the concept of "medical pluralism," that is, the use of so-called traditional, culturally bound notions of health and decision making in health care, and the concurrent acceptance of standard concepts of medicine and health care derived from Western cultural and the philosophic perspectives of the dominant culture. Also, clinicians should be mindful of the powerful effects of stereotyping, especially in circumstances where clinical decision making is occurring in hurry. Kagawa-Singer and Blackhall[13] have advanced an ABCDE mnemonic to assist clinicians in doing cultural assessments (**Table 1**).

Table 1
ABCDE cultural assessment model

Relevant Information	Questions and Strategies for the Health Care Provider
Attitudes of parents and families	Increase one's knowledge about the values, beliefs, and attitudes of the cultural group most frequent seen in your practice Assess their perspectives: What does your illness/sickness mean to you? Determine if the patient/family uses traditional health practices and for what problems Determine if the patient or family has positive or negative attitudes about a particular aspect of care (eg, discussion of or completion of advance directive documents)
Beliefs	Spiritual or religious strength sustain many people in times of distress. What is important for me to know about your faith or spiritual needs? How can we support your needs and practices? Where do you find your strength to make sense of what is happening to you?
Context (determine historical and political context of patient and family life)	Where were you born and raised? What language are you most comfortable using when talking about your health care? What are other important times in your life that might help us better understand your situation?
Decision-making style	Who is head of the family? How are decisions about health care made in your family?
Environment	Identify community resources

Adapted from Kagawa-Singer M, Backhall L. Negotiating cross-cultural issues at end of life. JAMA 2001;286(23):2993–3001.

How does one adopt and maintain an attitude of open-mindedness, curiosity, and respect for assessing the "3-state" reality of patients? Medical educators recommend that to improve knowledge, attitudes, and skills important to practicing truly holistic and personalized care, one should focus on "process oriented tools and concepts that will serve the practitioner well in communication and developing therapeutic alliances with all types of patients."[13,14]

A critical aspect of self-awareness and open-mindedness that promotes high-quality care is the realization that one is often blind to simple realities. An illustration of this is shown in **Box 2**. Most of us do not see all 6 of the "*Fs*" in this phrase until we deliberately stop and concentrate on the task.

The behavioral economist and Nobel Laureate, Daniel Kahneman, has pointed out that all people use 2 cognitive systems in addressing and solving problems.[14] System 1 is a so-called "fast" system of cognition, and System 2 is a so-called slower, more reflective system. System 1 cognition is good for making judgments, such as detecting if 1 object is more distant than another. System 2 cognitions are better for actions, such as organizing one's thought to "parking a narrow space." The simple question in **Box 3** illustrates the differences between System 1 and 2 thinking.

One of Kahneman's basic theses is that most people think they are operating in System 2, but are usually operating in system 1. He calls System 2 the "lazy controller" and has demonstrated that it is hard work to train System 2 to override the fast and intuitively based assumptions of System 1. Because of this, the most common answer to the "bat and baseball problem" in **Box 3** is answered quickly and incorrectly as $0.10. The correct answer is $0.05. Only when one slows down and reflects—even briefly—on the problem does one gain control over the error-prone actions of System 1.

There are many mental and cognitive strategies that one can use to minimize these types of errors in thinking. It is important to be aware that people use fast and slow cognitive styles to solve problems. One should use procedures which allow a slower, more reflective style of thinking, even when there is limited time.

In the context of trying to understand more fully and comprehensively the multiple identities, preference, and values of individuals experiencing serious illness, a useful strategy is to listen carefully and to encourage patients to tell stories of their illness.[15] It is vital to let sick persons tell their stories because illness unfolds in stories, which often gives patients a voice that has been rendered mute by the overwhelming presence of distress and suffering caused by illness.

Excellent palliative care clinicians have developed the skill of "narrative competence." This skill allows one to listen to the stories of patients and to gain a fuller and richer understanding of their experience—or as Rita Charon puts it: "the ability to adopt other's perspectives, to image and care about others' situations, to tolerate ambiguity and uncertainty... deepen the capacity to help the patients in our care."[16] Narrative competency is an important corrective for cultural blindness, lack of empathy, and inattentiveness to suffering. As Charon goes on to say, "With narrative methods, it is possible for practitioners... to focus their attention on the patient, to offer their whole selves toward healing, and to bear witness to those who suffer. By sharing our skill and our hope, we can join patients... as they reach toward the goals they choose in body, in self, and in life."[16]

Box 2
How many *Fs*?

"Finished files are the result of years of scientific study combined with the experience of many years."

Box 3
System 1 versus system 2 thinking: baseball and bat problem

A bat and ball cost $1.10.

The bat costs $1 more than the ball.

How much does the ball cost?

From Kahneman D. Thinking, fast and slow. New York: Farrar, Straus and Giroux; 2011.

SUMMARY

The journey to excellence in palliative care practice is to recognize the 3 identities of patients, to refine skills in assessment to understand these interrelated dimensions of personhood, and to hone the practices of caring to deliver truly comprehensive and personalized care. These practices require clinicians to first connect to persons with illness on a human–human level. Clinicians must train their "lazy controller" System 2 thinking to correctly process the complex and fast information that they encounter in all health care settings to avoid snap, error-filled judgments and stereotyping. Being fully present and engaged with patients, in addition to opening one's imagination to the sources of suffering that patients are experiencing, is critical to practicing high-quality palliative care. Finally, clinicians must encourage and elicit the story of the illness and the life of the person experiencing the illness by sharpening their narrative competency. This skill allows clinicians to practice the art of palliative care for their one person, with 3 identities and all of the complexities.

REFERENCES

1. Part of this section was previously published as Forward PR. Living with grief: diversity and end-of-life care. Washington, DC: Hospice Foundation of America; 2009. p. i–iii.
2. Kluckhohn C, Murray HA. Personality in nature, society, and culture. New York: A. A. Knopf; 1948. p. 35.
3. Crenshaw JL. The wisdom literature. In: Knight DA, Tucker GM, editors. The Hebrew Bible and its modern interpreters. 1985.
4. Culture. Attitudes and behaviors that are characteristic of a group or community. Learn more: what is cultural competence? Available at: http://minorityhealth.hhs.gov/omh Accessed January 15, 2015.
5. Verhey A. Reading the bible in the strange world of medicine. Grand Rapids (MI): William B. Eerdmans; 2003. p. 19–22.
6. Callahan D. Religion and the secularization of bioethics. Hastings Cent Rep 1990; 20:2–4.
7. Jennings B. The liberalism of life: bioethics in the face of biopower. Raritan 2003; 22(4):132–46.
8. A definition of irreversible coma. Report of the Ad Hoc Committee of the Harvard Medical School to examine the definition of brain death. JAMA 1968;205(6): 337–40.
9. President's Commission for the Study of Ethical Problems in Medicine and Biomedical and Behavioral Research (1981). Defining death: a report on the medical, legal and ethical issues in the determination of death. The President's Council on Bioethics web site: Available at: http://www.bioethics.gov/reports/past_commissions/defining_death.pdf. Accessed November 7, 2006.

10. Controversies in the Determination of Death. A white paper of the President's council on bioethics. Washington, DC; 2008. Available at: www.bioethics.gov. Accessed February 25, 2015.

11. 7th Circuit Court of Appeals Rules that SNF cannot respect patient's racial preferences - in Chaney v Plainfield Healthcare Center. Available at: http://www.hansonbridgett.com/Publications/pdf/~/media/7B4ED36B1B9B42FDBC78012ACED93F0B.pdf. Accessed February 25, 2015.

12. Jean Gilbert M, editor. Principles and recommended standards for cultural competence education of health care professionals. Los Angeles, CA: The California Endowment; 2003.

13. Kagawa-Singer M, Backhall L. Negotiating cross-cultural issues at end of life: "you got to go where he lives". JAMA 2001;286:2993.

14. Kahneman D. Thinking, fast and slow. New York: Farrar, Straus and Giroux; 2011. p. 45.

15. Charon R. Narrative medicine: honing the stories of illness. New York: Oxford University Press; 2008.

16. Charon R. A narrative medicine for pain. In: Daniel BC, John DL, Morris DB, editors. Narrative, pain, and suffering. Progress in pain research and management, vol. 34. Seattle (WA): IASP Press; 2005. p. 29–44.

International Palliative Care: Middle East Experience As a Model for Global Palliative Care

Ramzi R. Hajjar, MD, AGSF[a], Haris A. Charalambous, BM, MRCP, FRCR[b],
Lea Baider, PhD[c], Michael Silbermann, DMD, PhD[d],*

KEYWORDS

- Palliative care • Family • Illness • Treatment • Middle East • Cancer care • Aging
- Culture

KEY POINTS

- With the global shortage of palliative care (PC) specialists, it has become clear that care for elderly people with life-limiting illness cannot be delivered primarily by geriatricians or PC practitioners.
- In a culture in which family ties run deep, the offer of PC from an outsider is likely to be met with suspicion and distrust. The family bond in the Middle East may be stronger than in Western countries, but in contrast the emotional response to terminal illness may push families to request futile treatments, and physicians to comply. When PC is well developed and well understood, it provides a viable alternative to such extreme terminal measures.

INTRODUCTION

Palliative care (PC), as a specialty and model of care, is a recent construct in global health care, although the principle of alleviating suffering of the infirm is not novel. Modern medicine has seen great advances in diseases management and prevention, but until recently little attention had been given to supportive care of patients with cancer. This year alone, it is estimated that more than 8.2 million deaths will occur globally, of which 5.3 million (64.6%) will be in developing countries.[1] Moreover, in the near future, the number of elderly in developing countries is expected to increase dramatically, and with it the number of people needing PC. Experts estimate that 60%

[a] Geriatrics Medicine and Palliative Care Service, American University of Beirut Medical Center, Riad El Solh, Beirut 1107 2020, Lebanon; [b] Clinical Oncologist, The Bank of Cyprus Oncology Centre, 32 Acropoleus Avenue, Strovolos, Nicosia 2006, The Republic of Cyprus; [c] Psycho-Oncology Services, Assuta Medical Center, 20 Habarzel Street, Tel Aviv 69710, Israel; [d] The Middle East Cancer Consortium, 15 Kiryat Sefer str, Haifa 3467630, Israel
* Corresponding author.
E-mail address: cancer@mecc-research.com

Clin Geriatr Med 31 (2015) 281–294
http://dx.doi.org/10.1016/j.cger.2014.12.001
geriatric.theclinics.com

of all deaths could benefit from PC at some stage of the disease progression, but very few receive it.[2]

Over the past few decades, great progress has been made in the provision of PC in most parts of Europe, Canada, and Australia, and more recently a similar push was seen in the United States, where PC has been integrated into mainstream medicine. In contrast, PC in most developing countries remains underappreciated and poorly established, if available at all. The deficit is of such far-reaching impact that Singer and Bowman,[3] among others, argue that the quality end-of-life care should be viewed as a global public health and health systems problem. With an aging global population, this crisis is expected to worsen unless decisive steps are taken.

This article draws from our collective experience in introducing and promoting PC in the Middle East (ME). It examines the reasons why PC provision lags behind in most of the region's countries, and the challenges involved in overcoming this deficit. Real-life clinical vignettes are used to describe the cultural milieu that simultaneously hinders and welcomes PC, and the all-encompassing spiritual component present in most developing countries is examined. The Middle East and Northern Africa (MENA) region is used as a proxy model for global PC, because the generic parameters are grossly similar for most traditional families, even as specifics vary in style, solutions, resources, and constraints across different values and belief systems.[4] This article also favors the term PC rather than hospice in order to emphasize the need for symptom management throughout the trajectory of illness.

Palliative Care and the Developing World

Over the past century the world witnessed a demographic shift that has had profound impact on the practice of medicine and the delivery of health care. Toward the end of the nineteenth century, miasma theory gave way to the germ theory of disease, and micronutrient deficiencies were discovered as the cause of several debilitating illnesses. The introduction of aseptic surgery under general anesthesia, and the advancement of primary and preventive care, further played a major role in shaping the modern view of illness and health. These changes were the result of public health measures based on a deeper understanding of the pathophysiology of body structure and function, and the era of mechanization of medicine commenced.

As a result, many illnesses that were life limiting in the early 1900s became routinely treatable or preventable, and the number of elderly adults grew at an unprecedented rate. Life expectancy in westernized countries nearly doubled over the span of a century, and currently stands at around 80 years in most developed countries. Diseases that people used to die from last century became conditions they live with, and the medical establishment was not prepared to deal with the sequelae that chronic disease entails. Modern medicine not only prolonged life, but prolonged the dying trajectory as well. The proliferation of structured PC programs in parallel with aging societies in developed countries was not coincidental. The model of care that emerged to address the quality of life of patients with life-limiting illness served well the aging populations. Moreover, end-of-life palliation took on a renewed sense of urgency as causes of mortality shifted from acute illnesses (eg, infections, myocardial infarctions, nutritional deficiencies) to chronic degenerative disorders occurring late in life (eg, heart failure, dementia). The unintended consequence of longevity (mainly chronic illness) was a significant force in the evolution of PC conceptualization over the past 2 decades. Although the initial model of PC was based on patients with terminal cancers, it now embraces a broad spectrum of nonmalignant conditions.

In contrast, developing and low-income countries have not benefited from advances in medical sciences to the same extent as westernized countries. In some developing countries, life expectancy lags far behind that of developed countries because of the unrelenting burden of communicable diseases and malnutrition. In the second half of the twentieth century, global life expectancy increased from approximately 48 to 66 years, whereas it remains less than 60 years in many underdeveloped countries and has declined in 16 countries.[3,5] These regions have young populations and the causes of death (and hence end-of-life trajectories) differ markedly from those in developed countries. The global implication, and challenge, of this dichotomy is 2-fold: (1) end-of-life care strategies developed in westernized countries may not be suitable for developing countries where the context of death differs; and (2) a public health approach to PC is essential if global efforts are to be met with any measure of success.

The demographic shift toward aging will be particularly apparent over the next few decades in countries of the ME. Compared with developed countries, the population of the ME is young. The percentage of the population more than 65 years of age in MENA countries is estimated at 4.7% (of a total population of 336 million) according to the 2012 report of the World Bank.[6] The range varies from less than 2% in the United Arab Emirates (UAE) to approximately 10% in Lebanon. It is projected that, in 35 to 40 years, the youthful masses will move up the population pyramid and the geriatric population in the ME will surge. As in aging populations elsewhere, the fastest rate of growth will be in the very old. The World Health Organization (WHO) estimates that, from 2000 to 2050, the annual rate of growth of the population more than 65 years of age is projected to be 4% to 5%, and the average annual growth rate of the oldest old (85 years and older) will exceed 5% in 11 Arab countries.[7] In countries like Israel, Lebanon, and Cyprus, the proportion of elderly is already high and will double by the year 2050. Other countries, like Qatar, Kuwait, and UAE, should anticipate a 5-fold or greater increase in the proportion of their geriatric population and should allocate resources accordingly.

The ME is a diverse and heterogeneous region where politics and religion pervade most aspects of life, including health and health care. Countries in the ME can differ widely by religious practices, economic privileges, social structures, and cultural norms. Conventional Western medicine is generally adopted throughout the ME, but is implemented inconsistently and often practiced alongside faith healing and folk medicine. It is because of this diversity that the region serves well as a surrogate model in the discourse of international PC.

In addition to chronic disease, longevity also increases the lifetime cumulative risk for many types of cancer. Epidemiologic studies show that all-cause cancer incidence peaks around the age of 70 years. With a young population, the incidence of cancer in the ME is substantially lower compared with the US Surveillance, Epidemiology, and End Results (SEER).[8] However, over the next few decades, the incidence of cancer in the ME is expected to surge in parallel with the aging population. Registry data already indicate an increasing regional burden of cancer. Furthermore, cancer incidence projections are worsened by an indolent preventive care culture and casual approach to cancer screening, coupled with high prevalence of cancer-promoting behavior such as smoking and the adoption of a Western-style diet. Consequently, many cancers present at an advanced stage when symptoms alert to the presence of disease and the only reasonable intervention is PC.

Cancer survival rates vary greatly in different populations across the ME but generally fall short of Western standards.[9] The low cancer rate in the young population of developing countries is offset by worse outcome, and the overall impact of the disease is at least as great as in developed countries. Global cancer statistics show that, although the overall cancer incidence rates in the developing world are half those seen in the developed world in both sexes, cancer mortalities are similar.[10] The WHO argues that any governmental cancer program, particularly in low-income countries, should address 4 key components of care: prevention, early detection, treatment, and PC. The last component has been notably missing from most programs in developing countries. Only with comprehensive national policies that combine promotion of healthy lifestyle choices, mass screening, and access to effective treatment will the increasing prevalence of cancer in the ME be combated. In addition, to reduce the psychosocial impact of cancer, education, stigma reduction, and PC services will be necessary.

An important distinction between PC and terminal cancer care must be made at this point. Longevity and the resulting surge in chronic disease mean that an increasing proportion of PC effort is being allocated to noncancerous ailments. A global survey conducted by the WHO in 2011 estimated that only 34% of adults in need of PC had cancer.[5] PC is no longer primarily the domain of terminal cancer care, but in the ME the distinction is largely lost. Since March 2011, the American University of Beirut Medical Center has offered inpatient PC under the direction of the sole certified PC and geriatric specialist (coauthor RH). Over the course of 3 years, 123 patients were referred for end-of-life care. Most were elderly (n = 111; 90%), and 91 (74%) had malignant conditions (Hajjar RR, unpublished data; Presented at the Annual Meeting of the American Geriatric Society – Special interest Group on Ethnogeriatrics, 2013. Grapevine, TX). Most patients who did not have cancer had end-stage Parkinson disease and dementia (n = 22; 18%). This pattern of use is prevalent in developing countries, and is in contrast with patterns in the United States, where approximately two-thirds of hospice enrollees have nonmalignant diagnoses according to the Medicare Hospice Benefits report. In the ME and other developing countries worldwide, this budding specialty has little utility outside the realm of oncology, and continues to be stigmatized by association with the dying patients with cancer. However, the pattern of PC use is likely to change as public awareness and acceptance become more prevalent.

BRIDGING THE CULTURAL CHASM

Multiculturalism in the social and behavioral sciences has recently gained profile owing to studies of in-crisis families facing grief, illness, and death.[11,12] The multicultural dimension recognizes the value of cultural differentiation in the assessment-of-care process, as family needs are accommodated throughout the progression of illness and ultimately death.[13] Chronic illness and end-of-life care among the elderly should be conceptualized in terms of cultural values, social milieu, religious beliefs, and family perceptions. Traditional cultural values and long-established norms of behavior recognize intergenerational processes as an attempt to preserve family continuity and stability in times of crisis.[14] Cancer and other serious illnesses never occur in isolation. A specific family dynamic exists, with its accompanying strong cultural tradition and recurring intergenerational relationships.[15] This dynamic is particularly evident with life-threatening illnesses, in which issues of appraisal and significance assume vital importance for family adaptation.[16,17]

Culture is more significant than mere tradition grounded in intergenerational norms. It extends to the fundamental way in which the world is perceived.[3] Furthermore, attitudes toward end-of-life care are specific to particular cultures, societies, and periods.[18] When facing people of different cultural backgrounds, the unspoken assumptions can be so different that constructive end-of-life discussions could be ineffective or break down altogether.[3]

An important tenet of Western medical ethics is the deep-rooted belief that health care decisions are best made by the individual experiencing the illness after full disclosure. Involving other persons in the discussion, even family members, must only proceed with the explicit consent of the patient. In many non-Western cultures, including the ME, this strict adhesion to autonomy is not only discounted, but occasionally viewed as disruptive to patient care. The extended family or community support system is perceived as vital in disclosing information and decision making. Central to understanding the responses of elderly patients with cancer to their illness is the appreciation of the role of family values.[19] In the ME, the cultural code for the position of the elder within the family is strongly influenced by the force of traditional values and stratification norms. This code includes the boundaries that regulate proximity and separateness (inclusion or exclusion of the other), boundaries that regulate hierarchy (gender and generation power balances), values associated with personal individuation and family connectedness, and communication styles with the health care provider.[20] The last of these is of particular significance to the PC practitioner, who must understand and accede to local and individual custom of conduct if guidance is to be effective. The following 2 clinical scenarios demonstrate these principles.

Aabidah: a Narrative of Hope and Grief

Ibrahim was 70 years old. His medical condition in 2010 included the diagnosis of lung cancer (small cell undifferentiated carcinoma) and hepatic metastases. He was hospitalized with pneumonia for the last 3 weeks of his illness and died the day after his return home.

Patient background

Aabidah is his 56-year-old wife and caregiver. They have 6 children aged 17 to 28 years, most of them married. Ibrahim has 4 brothers and 2 sisters, who live together with their widowed father in a small village in the north. The family operates a clothing store business in which all the male family members are employed.

Sequence of events

Aabidah spent the last 3 weeks of Ibrahim's illness, while he was sedated and receiving oxygen, entirely in the hospital. Much of the time, Ibrahim's room was filled with elder male family members, many of whom prayed at his bedside. At the family's request, the hospital bed was turned toward Mecca. Aabidah did not request help from the nurses; she washed Ibrahim, attended to his needs, and prepared his food every day, regardless of the fact that he was being fed intravenously.

At the end of 3 weeks, the physician discussed Ibrahim's imminent death with the male members of the family. Their response was to request his release from the hospital in order to return Ibrahim to his home. The medical staff asked for permission to speak to Ibrahim and his wife regarding the risks and consequences of leaving the hospital, but the family categorically opposed such intervention. The elder male members of the family emphasized their sole responsibility for resolving medical issues. In addition, they clarified 2 fundamental convictions: God's determination of the individual's voyage into another life, and the submission of women to the elder's decision.

The day after he arrived home, Ibrahim died in his bed surrounded by his brothers and the rest of the men in the family. Aabidah covered herself in black, silent in her weeping and sorrow. Just before Ibrahim's departure for home, Aabidah had visited and embraced me (LB). She placed a piece of paper in my hand, on which was written: "Indeed, I am to die…just as death is certain, so is the resurrection of the dead. Qur'an, 2:153. I will wait for Ibrahim…always. God is always in our soul. Aabidah." (From the diary of L. Baider.)

Abraham: An Enduring Hope

Abraham was diagnosed with prostate cancer in 1993 and bone metastasis in 1999. He died in 2005.

Patient background

Abraham was born in 1923 in Iraq, and immigrated to Israel with his family in 1930. Abraham had 5 children and 19 grandchildren, aged 10 to 30 years. His parents, who died when Abraham was young, came from a highly religious Orthodox Jewish family. From a young age, Abraham was involved in religious studies and eventually became a rabbi. His first wife died of cancer and in 1995 he married his second wife, who was 13 years his junior.

Sequence of events

Abraham's wife was totally devoted to him and his family. Abraham was a firm believer that he would be cured as a result of direct prayers to God. Aside from a younger and less religious daughter, Abraham's family encouraged this belief. The daughter was at odds with the rest of the family, not accepting that their "lies" sheltered her father, or agreeing with their passive attitude. However, the family managed to overcome her rebellion by accusing her of selfishness and arousing her guilty feelings.

Physicians, who held a similar religious view as Abraham, accepted the patient's silence and did not communicate with him. The medical team offered little besides strong opiates for pain. In 2003, the family requested a wheelchair to facilitate Abraham's sharing meals and additional time with family members. However, Abraham did not cooperate with this suggestion, and continued to believe he was alone and misunderstood.

Abraham's home became a center of perpetual activity, with visitors bringing food, helping with caregiving, and participating in all-male prayer. No separation was made between the healthy and the ill. Both the home hospice and the health care team went along with patient's perception of the illness (denial). Nevertheless, despite (or because of) the perpetual noise, silence prevailed in Abraham's spirit. Within dreams and hopes, the patient only whispered to God. His only truth, his credo, was in the benevolence and compassion of his God. Abraham died in unspoken stillness. The prayers and sounds did not hinder his own dialogue with God. (From the diary of L. Baider.)

These two clinical stories highlight the patient and family similarity of responses toward illness and death. In one case it is the silence of the caretaker, in the other, the silence of the patient. Both cases depict a pattern of conduct that is considered the norm in the ME but conflicts with established Western standards of care.

Cancer: Intertwining of Belief Systems

The trajectory of chronic illness adapts itself to the life course of elderly patients and contributes intimately to the development and solidification of particular rituals. Illness enters into the daily narrative of the family and it becomes accepted practice for elder family members to contribute significantly to any decision-making process and to assume total caregiving responsibilities.[12]

Collective decision making is the norm in traditional culture, often clashing with the value of autonomy and individual prerogative regarding medical decisions.[21] These core/traditional values may create a dilemma for the health care provider attempting to involve the patient in the treatment plan. In collective decision making, health and sickness are restricted to family models of resolution, because older male family members become the spokespersons on behalf of the family.[22] These elder family members become the primary participants in decision making for the patients.

According to Islamic and Orthodox Jewish religious systems of law, the family is the basic unit charged with responsibility for decisions regarding treatment and disclosure. Religious families are usually reluctant to disclose the diagnosis of a terminal illness, believing that this may lead to emotional trauma, premature death, or both. Such reticence is especially true of a patient at the terminal stage of illness. Hope for prolonged life may be undermined by the knowledge that the patient cannot be cured.[23,24]

The obligations to preserve life and for nondisclosure or partial disclosure are not perceived as contradictory. In some traditional cultures, talking openly about death with an elderly person is not acceptable. Such discussion is considered disrespectful, bad luck, or the basis for loss of hope,[20–22] and may accelerate the dying process. Many cultures actively protect dying family members from being informed of their prognosis.[25] For example, some may request that patients not be informed of their imminent death out of concern for the patient's loss of hope, and the belief that only God can decide a person's fate.

This religious perspective can give meaning to the dying process and is at the core of differences between traditional and Western medicine. Western medicine is largely centered on objective reasoning and scientific principles. In essence, this is as much a cultural construction as any other belief system used in developing countries. Disease is perceived as an entity to be controlled, and death is viewed as a failure of medical care. Consequently, many patients expect medical solutions throughout the disease trajectory, and futile aggressive treatments at end of life can become extreme. Western terminology such as to battle with cancer and fight the disease reflect this attitude, and can become an added source of distress as the illness inexorably takes its natural course and patients perceive a sense of failure. In contrast, non-Western societies tend to perceive illness and death in a much broader manner. They accept death as a natural process and normal phase of life, even as they use florid belief systems to explain it. Some cultures believe illness is a separate entity brought about by external influences such as envy (the evil eye), witchcraft, or as retribution. These traditional belief systems can be powerful, and must be integrated into the PC plan of action. The concept of illness as a punishment from God or some other deity for patient or family indiscretions is observed in some traditional religious cultures. Suffering is then viewed as compensation and a rite of passage. Although this belief is not prevalent, it must be recognized because it is not discussed openly and may have a direct bearing on the acceptance of PC services at end of life.

For some religious Muslims, the taboo of discussing death with the family is facilitated by religious leaders. In extreme cases, the spiritual leader is given authority for medical decisions and becomes the surrogate decision maker. Inevitably, this hinders the physician's ability to communicate directly with the patient, because decisions are made directly by extended family members or religious authorities. Family culture suggests that members who have established strong religious beliefs are particularly likely to use religious explanations that preserve and reinforce their existing beliefs.[25] It is essential for the health care provider to have a clear understanding and recognition of the unique influence of culture and religion on family behavior, attitudes, preferences, and decisions regarding end-of-life care.

Health care professionals have developed and clung to their own culture, set of traditions, and belief systems, influenced and nurtured by their intergenerational family history. In the encounter with families of diverse religious cultures, clinicians must pursue a broader understanding, rather than the preconceived notions of what the family is or should be. This attitude will allow new kinds of debate regarding family care, health, and autonomy, and novel concepts of therapeutic processes. In so doing, controversy and quandaries will assume new qualities and new challenges.

BEYOND THE CULTURAL CHALLENGE

Palliative medicine is still in its infancy in the ME. There is abundant information as to why so many people with life-limiting illnesses do not receive adequate pain relief and symptom management. Experts estimate that 60% of those who die each year require PC, but a very small proportion of them receive it.[2] The 4 stages of PC development according to the classification of Wright and Clark[26] are described in **Table 1**.[27] Most ME countries are in the early development stage (capacity building). Syria has only recently entered the early capacity building stage, whereas the Palestinian territories have made respectable progress within geopolitical restraints. Many challenges must be overcome before PC is integrated into mainstream medicine and comfortably accepted by patients and health care providers. Obstacles to appropriate PC and pain management can be classified into 3 broad categories:

- Lack of trained personnel.
- Lack of government health policies for PC program development, including limited resources and investment in community hospice programs and low per-capita health expenditure

Table 1
Stages of PC development

Stage 1	Stage 2	Stage 3	Stage 4
No Services	**Capacity Building**	**Localized Provision**	**Approaching Integration**
Palestine, Syria	Most ME Countries	Jordan, Saudi Arabia	Israel, Cyprus
	Awareness of PC needs	Initial capacity building	Capacity building and localized services
	Being registered with key organizations; eg, EAPC/WHO/MECC	Local campaigning and publicity	Regular campaigning and publicity countrywide
	International links with other hospice/PC service providers	Services set up (ie, home care) and funding established	Range of providers and service types
	Conference participation	Government legislation in progress (NCCP to include PC)	Broad awareness of PC needs
	Visits to hospice-PC organizations	Opioids available	Some integration with mainstream health providers
	Education and training (visiting teams/ overseas training)	Training within hospice organization plus external training courses	Opioid and PC health policy/legislation agreed
	Preparation of development strategy; ie, lobbying of policy makers/health ministries for PC to be part of the National Cancer Control Plan	Developing academic links	Established education centers
		Developing research activity	Academic links and development of core curricula for undergraduate and postgraduate training
			Research activity: national and international publications

Abbreviations: EAPC, European Association of Palliative Care; MECC, Middle East Cancer Consortium; NCCP, National Cancer Control Program.

- Poor availability of opiates and other essential medications

Until recently, little attention had been given to the undergraduate and postgraduate training of health care professionals on pain management and end-of-life care in developing countries. Principles of PC had not been included in the licensing examinations of doctors or nurses, and many health care professionals did not view symptom management as a goal in itself. Only recently have medical schools throughout the ME introduced end-of-life instruction to their curricula. All medical and nursing schools now offer some form of instruction on death and dying, but this is only a recent development and often provides nominal exposure at best. Formal training in PC continues to be overlooked by most training programs. Even well-intentioned programs do not have the human resources to achieve this goal.

One of the largest obstacles to the provision of good PC and pain management is the lack of well-trained health care workers. Many do not have an adequate understanding of PC, and equate it with giving up. It is often initiated late in the trajectory of the disease, and is shrouded in various myths and misconceptions related to accelerating the dying process. Most providers have not been adequately trained in the proper use of opioid medications, and have misplaced fear of causing addiction or respiratory suppression. The global shortage of qualified providers is a system problem that will not be easy to overcome. The American Academy of Hospice and Palliative Medicine (AAHPM) commissioned a study in 2010 to assess just this problem.[28] PC physicians were identified by board certification or membership in the AAHPM, and were compared with the number of full-time providers needed to staff the current number of hospice-based and hospital-based PC programs at appropriate levels. The conservative estimated shortfall was at least 2787 full-time physicians, or approximately 6000 palliative medicine physicians given the proportion of time each physician devotes to PC. This current estimate did not factor in the unmet need for outpatient specialty PC clinics, or the sizable number of patients in need of PC but still unregistered in programs; nor does it address the future growth of PC needs in an aging population, and this is in the United States. Very few fellowship-trained PC physicians move to developing countries, where the need is so much greater. Lupu[28] concludes that the current capacity of fellowship programs is insufficient to fill the shortage.

Another serious deficit of the education system is the attitude of professionals toward death and dying. The inability or refusal of clinicians to discuss terminal issues with patients and their caregivers has become an accepted model of care resulting in unnecessary anguish and suffering. Aside from the cultural impediment, this deficiency is a result of poor training. In a survey of 1205 practicing Lebanese nurses and physicians, only 19.1% of physicians reported informing terminally ill patients about their diagnoses.[29] One-third of physicians (33.3%) said they do not inform patients of the diagnosis, and 37.7% said they only disclose information to patients if the families wished for them to do so. In another study of 126 medical students, 3 barriers to disclosing bad news were reported: fear of causing more distress to patients, family interference, and physician uncertainty.[30] Only 14% of students were given the opportunity to observe a senior physician disclose bad news to patients. In this instance, deficits in communication skills, empathy, and confidence are deficits of the education system.

One way of assessing the current status of PC provision in any country is opioid consumption, measured as morphine equivalence consumed per capita per year. This metric has been put forward by the WHO as a universal health care indicator for PC. Although it is a surrogate and not a direct measure of quality of care, it is a measurable objective indicator and reflects progress in PC intervention and policy. A large variation is seen in opiate availability and use between individual countries of the ME (**Tables 2–4**). Compared with global use and neighboring Mediterranean

Table 2
Availability of opioids in the ME according to International Association of Hospice and Palliative Care (IAHPC) lists

	Cyprus	Egypt	Israel	Jordan	Lebanon	Oman	Palestine	Syria	Turkey
Codeine, oral	✓	X	✓		✓	✓	✓	✓	✓
Morphine, oral immediate release	✓	✓	✓	✓	X	✓	X	✓	X
Morphine, oral controlled release	✓	✓	✓	✓	✓	✓	✓	✓	✓
Injectable morphine	✓	✓	✓	✓	✓	✓	✓	✓	✓/X[a]
Oxycodone, oral immediate release	✓	X	✓		X	X	X	✓	X
Methadone, oral immediate release	✓	X	✓		X	X	X	X	X
Fentanyl, transdermal patch	✓	✓	✓		✓	✓	✓	✓	✓

[a] Limited availability of only 10-mg ampoules.
Data from Silberman M, Arnaout M, Daher M, et al. Palliative cancer care in Middle Eastern countries: accomplishments and challenges 2012. Ann Oncol Suppl 2012;3:15–28; and Cleary J, Silbermann M, Scholten W, et al. Formulary availability and regulatory barriers to accessibility of opioids for cancer pain in the Middle East: a report from the Global Opioid Policy Initiative (GOPI). Ann Oncol 2013;24 (Suppl 11):xi54.

countries, it is clear that regional use is suboptimal, with the exception of Israel. On a global scale, differences in opioid consumption are often caused by availability problems and excessive regulatory restrictions. Other barriers include both physician and patient factors,[31] notably fear of addiction and respiratory suppression. A recent study

Table 3
Regulatory restrictions to accessibility of opioids in the ME

	Cyprus	Egypt	Israel	Lebanon	Oman	Palestine	Syria
Requirement for registration of patients to receive opioids	—	Yes	—	Yes	Yes	Yes	Yes
Requirement for physicians to have a license to prescribe opioids	—	Yes	—	Yes	Yes	Yes	Yes
Requirement for duplicate prescriptions or use of special prescription forms	Yes	Yes	—	Yes	Yes	Yes	Yes
Limited prescription duration	—	Yes	—	—	—	Yes	—
No pharmacist authority to correct prescription	Yes	Yes	Yes	Yes	—	Yes	Yes
Limitations on dispensing sites	—	Yes	—	Yes	Yes	Yes	Yes
No emergency prescribing or nonmedical prescribing	Yes	Yes	Yes	Yes	Yes	Yes	Yes
Use of stigmatizing terms for opioid analgesics in regulations	—	—	Yes	Yes	—	Yes	—

Adapted from Cleary J, Silbermann M, Scholten W, et al. Formulary availability and regulatory barriers to accessibility of opioids for cancer pain in the Middle East: a report from the Global Opioid Policy Initiative (GOPI). Ann Oncol 2013;24 (Suppl 11):xi55; with permission.

Table 4
Opiate use for select Mediterranean and ME countries in 2001 and 2011 and comparison with the United States and global consumption

Country	2001 Morphine Equivalence (mg/person)	2011 Morphine Equivalence (mg/person)	Increase in Morphine Equivalence (mg/person)	Increase in Morphine Equivalence (%)
Cyprus	12.2	35.1	22.9	187.7
Egypt	0.7	1.0	0.3	42.8
Israel	150.2	154.8	4.6	3.1
Jordan	9.2	24.3	15.1	164.1
Lebanon	5.4	4.9	−0.5	−9.2
Oman	1.8	3.9	2.1	116.7
Syria	1.1	3.8	2.7	245.5
Turkey	3.8	12.2	8.4	221.1
Italy	75.9	169.4	93.5	123.2
Greece	48.6	115.0	66.4	136.6
United States	542.8	749.8	207.0	38.1
Global	39.3	61.7	22.4	57.0

Data from Pain and Policy Studies Group, University of Wisconsin, Madison WI. Available at: http://www.painpolicy.wisc.edu. Accessed October 26, 2014.

found that regulatory restrictions (and hence opioid availability) are a significant barrier in countries of the ME.[32] Only 2 countries (Cyprus and Israel) had access to all 7 essential drugs listed by the WHO and International Association of Hospice and Palliative Care.

THE WAY FORWARD

In order to accelerate recent global efforts to promote PC as a viable model of care and patient right, efforts by qualified individuals must be sustained on many fronts. A bottom-up approach should target young health care providers in order to generate a cadre of culturally sensitive health professionals who in turn act as role models and push for quality end-of-life care and policy reform. Simultaneously, a top-down approach is essential to lobby governmental organizations to amend legislation regarding opioid availability and resource allocation. In societies deeply entrenched in tradition and rituals, a trusted third party may best fill this role. The Middle East Cancer Consortium (MECC) is such an organization, and has had significant impact on promoting PC in MENA countries.

It is thought that the main obstacle in providing quality PC and pain management globally and in the ME is the lack of knowledge and training of health care professionals in PC and the poor opportunities to address those deficiencies through training. In view of this, MECC under the guidance of Professor Michael Silbermann has adopted the mission of training professionals in the region through individualized courses in PC in different countries, regional workshops, and exchange programs with PC institutions in the United States. MECC works in conjunction with the Oncology Nursing Society (ONS) and the American Society of Clinical Oncology (ASCO), and is supported by the National Cancer Institute. The regional benefit resulting from efforts of the MECC and other organization such as the International Association of Hospice and Palliative Care (IAHPC) over the past 10 years has been tangible. In a recent needs assessment, a convenience sample of 776 health care professionals from 14 MENA countries was surveyed.[33,34] Two encouraging key findings were that more than 90% of respondents were familiar with the concept of PC, and that pain relief and symptom management are offered to 70% of patients with cancer in the region. The biggest barriers to providing optimal care were lack of community awareness, lack of staff training, and shortage of PC beds and services. Fear of using opioids and lack of availability were ranked low on the list of barriers.

In countries with limited resources, local customs and nontraditional resources can be used creatively to fill the need. The culture of the ME is not receptive to placing elderly patients in nursing homes. This culture provides a unique opportunity to have good community PC teams to help families to look after patients at home, particularly because continuous live-in support in the form of domestic workers is affordable to middle-income families. The role of the PC nurse would be to educate the caretakers, and to provide reassurance as they look after their ailing relatives. This provides the basis for the proposal that the family can function as a PC unit at home.

SUMMARY

With the global shortage of PC specialists, it has become clear that care for older people with life-limiting illness cannot be delivered primarily by geriatricians or PC practitioners. The role of these clinicians is to help all those who deliver care become more adept in the principles and practice of PC medicine.

In a culture in which family ties run deep, the offer of PC from an outsider is likely to be met with suspicion and distrust. The family bond in the ME may be stronger than in Western countries, but in contrast the emotional response to terminal illness may push families to request futile treatments, and physicians to comply. When PC is well developed and well understood, it provides a viable alternative to such extreme terminal measures.

REFERENCES

1. GLOBOCAN 2012. IARC 2013. Available at: http://globocan.iarc.fr/old/factsheet. asp. Accessed October 1, 2014.
2. Human Rights Watch. Global state of pain treatment - access to medicines and palliative care. New York: Human Rights Watch; 2011. Available at: www.hrw. org/sites/default/files/reports/hhr0511W. Accessed October 1, 2014.
3. Singer PA, Bowman KW. Quality end-of-life care: a global perspective. BMC Palliat Care 2002;1(1):4.
4. Jean-Pierre P, Fiscella K, Griggs J. Race-ethnicity-based concerns over understanding cancer diagnosis and treatment. JAMA 2010;102:184–9.
5. World Health Organization. Worldwide palliative care alliance: global atlas of palliative care at the end of life. In: Connor SR, Bermedo MC, editors. London: Worldwide Palliative Care Alliance; 2014. p. 10–25.
6. The World Bank annual report, vol. 1. Washington, DC: Main Report; 2012. Available at: https://openknowledge.worldbank.org/handle/10986/11844. Accessed September 8, 2014.
7. Economic and Social Affairs of the United Nations Secretariat. World Population Prospects: the 2006 Revision. Available at: http://www.un.org/esa/population/ unpop.htm. Accessed August 1, 2014.
8. Freedman LS, Edwards BK, Ries LAG, et al, editors. Cancer incidence in four member countries (Cyprus, Egypt, Israel, and Jordan) of the Middle East Cancer

Consortium (MECC) compared with US SEER. Bethesda (MD): National Cancer Institute; 2006. NIH Pub. No. 06–5873.

9. Silberman M, Arnaout M, Daher M, et al. Palliative cancer care in Middle Eastern countries: accomplishments and challenges. Ann Oncol 2012; 23(Suppl 3):15–28.

10. Jemal A, Bray F, Center MM, et al. Global cancer statistics. CA Cancer J Clin 2011;61:69–90.

11. Kagawa-Singer M, Backhall L. Negotiating cross-cultural issues at end of life. JAMA 2010;286(23):2993–3001.

12. Kagawa-Singer M, Valdez D, Yu M. Cancer, culture and health disparities: time to chart a new course? CA Cancer J Clin 2010;60:12–39.

13. Coolen PR. Cultural relevance in end-of-life care. EthnoMedicine 2012.

14. Kline M, Huff R. 2nd edition. Health promotion in multicultural populations, vol. Los Angeles (CA); London; New Delhi (India); Singapore: SAGE; 2007. Chapter 1–3.

15. Sparling TC. Caring for Fatima. J Clin Oncol 2006;24:2589–91.

16. Baider L. Cancer in different cultural context: how is the family affected? EONS Newsletter 2007;72:515–22.

17. Sluzki CE. The pathway between conflict and reconciliation: co-existence as an evolutionary process. Transcult Psychiatry 2010;47:55–69.

18. Bowman KW. Culture, ethics and the biodiversity crisis of Central Africa. Advances in Applied Biodiversity 2001;2:167–74.

19. Baider L. Cancer and the family: the myth of words and silences. Pediatr Hematol Oncol 2010;32:533–57.

20. Giger J, Davidhizar R, Fordham P. Multi-cultural and multi-ethnic considerations and advanced directives: developing cultural competency. J Cult Divers 2006; 13(1):3–9.

21. Huff R, Kline M. Health promotion in the context of culture. In: Kline M, Huff R, editors. Health promotion in multicultural populations. 2nd edition. Los Angeles (CA); London; New Delhi (India); Singapore: SAGE; 2007. p. 3–22.

22. Searight H, Gafford J. Cultural diversity at the end of life: issues and guidelines for family physicians. Am Fam Physician 2005;71(3):515–22.

23. Jones RB, Pearson J, Cawsey AL. Effect of different forms of information produced for cancer patients on their use of information: randomized trial. BMJ 2006;332:942–6.

24. Baider L. Communication about illness: a family narrative. Support Care Cancer 2008;16:607–11.

25. Carteret M. Cultural group guides. Dimensions of culture cross-cultural communications for healthcare professionals. 2012. Available at: http://www.dimensionsofculture.com. Accessed October 1, 2014.

26. Wright M, Clark D. Hospice and palliative care in Africa: a review of development and challenges. Lancaster, UK: Oxford University Press; 2006.

27. Bingley A, Clark D. A comparative view of palliative care development in six countries represented by the Middle East Cancer Consortium (MECC). J Pain Symptom Manage 2009;37:287–96.

28. Lupu D. Estimates of current hospice and palliative medicine physician workforce shortage. J Pain Symptom Manage 2010;40:899–911.

29. Huijer H, Dimassi H. Palliative care in Lebanon: knowledge, attitudes and practices of physicians and nurses. J Med Liban 2007;55:121–8.

30. Antoun J, Saab BR. A culturally sensitive audiovisual package to teach breaking bad news in a Lebanese setting. Med Teach 2010;32(10):868–9.

31. Charalambous H, Protopapa E, Gavrielidou D, et al. Physicians' prescribing habits for cancer pain in Cyprus. Ann Oncol 2012;23(Suppl 3):79–83. Available at: http://www.ncbi.nlm.nih.gov/pubmed/22628422.http://www.ncbi.nlm.nih.gov/pubmed?term=Charalambous%20H%5BAuthor%5D&cauthor=true&cauthor_uid=22628422.

32. Cleary J, Silbermann M, Scholten W, et al. Formulary availability and regulatory barriers to accessibility of opioids for cancer pain in the Middle East: a report from the Global Opioid Policy Initiative (GOPI). Ann Oncol 2013;24(Suppl 11): xi51–9.

33. Silberman M, Fink RM, Min SJ, et al. Evaluating palliative care needs in Middle Eastern countries. J Palliat Med 2015;18:1–8.

34. Pain and Policy Studies Group. University of Wisconsin. Available at: http://www.painpolicy.wisc.edu/country/profiles. Accessed October 26, 2014.

Emergency Medicine and Palliative Care

Derrick S. Lowery, MD[a], Tammie E. Quest, MD[b],*

KEYWORDS

- Emergency • Resuscitation • Hospice • Stabilization • Critical care

KEY POINTS

- The emergency department cares for patients during sentinel events in their care trajectory.
- Emergency clinicians should not delay hospice or palliative care referrals in patients for whom there can be a benefit.
- Palliative care consultation services can integrate with the emergency department in a collaborative manner to improve access to hospice and palliative care services.

INTRODUCTION: THE NATURE OF THE PROBLEM

The primary focus in emergency medicine (EM) is the identification and stabilization of acute conditions with an emphasis on rapidly intervening and initiating necessary procedures and treatments. However, the emergency department (ED) has evolved beyond this to serve as the gateway to the resources of the hospital in many situations and is the entrance point for patients who have presented to the hospital in distress. The ED is a critical place of care delivery for seriously ill patients and families in need of a response to physical, spiritual, and psychological distress. For some, unfortunately, it is the site of their death.

Despite the perceived need, the evidence is lacking regarding the prevalence of seriously ill patients in need of palliative care support in the emergency setting.[1] In Ontario, more than 81% of patients with cancer visited an ED in the last 6 months of life, with 34% of the visits in the last 2 weeks of life. In the last 2 weeks of life, 70% of the visits resulted in a hospital admission. The most common reason for visits include pain and symptom management as well as failure of caregivers to cope with distress at home.[2] Nearly 400,000 persons will die in a US ED.[3] Up to 25% of patient

[a] Emory University School of Medicine, 1462 Clifton Road, Suite 302, Atlanta, GA 30322, USA;
[b] Department of Emergency Medicine, Emory Palliative Care Center, Emory School of Medicine, 1462 Clifton Road, Suite 302, Atlanta, GA 30322, USA
* Corresponding author.
E-mail address: tquest@emory.edu

Clin Geriatr Med 31 (2015) 295–303
http://dx.doi.org/10.1016/j.cger.2015.01.009
0749-0690/15/$ – see front matter Published by Elsevier Inc.

geriatric.theclinics.com

visits with advanced cancer may have been avoidable.[4] Palliative care approaches and interventions in the ED may present an opportunity to initiate optimal physical, spiritual, and psychological support. Consistently, studies that assess the palliative care needs in cancer and noncancer populations show that patients and families can benefit from physical, spiritual, psychological, and social support during the emergency crisis.

The ED often serves as a key branch point from which health care plans are determined. Patients present to the ED when they have acute distressing symptoms, such as pain or dyspnea, that their care support system cannot meet; when they do not know how to access the health care system; when they lack access to primary care or have been lost to follow-up; when they require diagnostic interventions like advanced imaging; or when they require acute interventions, such as intravenous fluids or medications. Despite optimal palliative care, patients will present to the ED when their distressing condition cannot be managed. The ED stop on patients' health care journey makes the ED an area ripe with opportunity for initiation of palliative care and continued linkage to support when patients are receiving comprehensive palliative care services.[5] Seventy-seven percent of patients who visited the ED during the last month of life were hospitalized, and 68% ultimately died in the acute care setting, demonstrating an opportunity to identify and redirect these patients to a setting that may be more in alignment with their goals.[6]

Despite this opportunity, historically, palliative care with its emphasis on multiple domains of comfort (physical, emotional, spiritual, and social) has been considered by some as incongruous with the culture of EM.

Included in these distressed patients are people with life-limiting diseases, such as terminal cancer, severe congestive heart failure, dementia, or renal failure, who are presenting to the ED with the goal of symptom management. A disconnect between the patients' goals and the provider's goals may then exist when the ED provider is working on stabilization, evaluation, and intervention of an acute event while the patients' goal is one of palliation of their distressing condition. Recognition of this possible disconnect is the first step necessary to take advantage of this checkpoint on a patient's journey with the health care system.[7–9]

The importance of palliative care in EM has been demonstrated when the American College of Emergency Physicians (ACEP) participated in the American Board of Internal Medicine's Choosing Wisely campaign in 2012. ACEP chose a palliative medicine domain for emergency providers to implement.

Don't delay engaging available palliative and hospice care services in the ED for patients likely to benefit. Palliative care is medical care that provides comfort and relief of symptoms for patients who have chronic and/or incurable diseases. Hospice care is palliative care for those patients in the final few months of life. Emergency physicians should engage patients who present to the ED with chronic or terminal illnesses, and their families, in conversations about palliative care and hospice services. Early referral from the ED to hospice and palliative care services can benefit select patients resulting in both improved quality and quantity of life.[10]

THERAPEUTIC OPTIONS

Determining the prevalence of palliative care needs in the ED is largely unknown.[1] However, general guidelines regarding patients that might benefit from both primary and/or subspecialty palliative care interventions in the ED have been identified (**Table 1**). Primary palliative care skills critical to the practice of the ED have also been identified (**Box 1**). Rapid assessments of the clinical scenario with key elements

Table 1
Criteria for initiation of a palliative care assessment

	Patient Presents with a Life-Limiting or Life-Threatening Condition[a]
Primary Criteria[b]	
1. The surprise question	Not surprised if patient died within 12 mo
2. Bounce-backs	More than one ED visit or hospital admission for same condition within the past several months
3. Difficult-to-control symptoms	Moderate to severe physical or psychological symptom intensity
4. Complex care requirements	Functional dependency; complex home support for ventilator/antibiotics
5. Functional decline	Feeding intolerance or unintended decline in weight (eg, failure to thrive)
Secondary Criteria[c]	
1. Admission from long-term care facility	
2. Elderly patients, cognitively impaired, with acute hip fracture	
3. Metastatic or locally advanced incurable cancer	
4. Chronic home oxygen use	
5. Out-of-hospital cardiac arrest	
6. Current or past hospice or palliative care intervention	
7. Limited social support (eg, family stress, caregiver distress, chronic mental illness)	
8. No history of completing an advance care planning document or having a discussion	

[a] Any disease or condition that is known to be life limiting (eg, dementia, chronic renal failure, metastatic cancer, or cirrhosis) or that has a high chance of leading to death (eg, sepsis, multiorgan failure, or major trauma).
[b] Primary criteria: global indicators that represent the minimum standard of care that hospitals should use to screen patients at risk for unmet palliative care needs.
[c] Secondary criteria: indicators of a high likelihood of unmet palliative care needs that should be incorporated into a systems-based approach to patient identification if possible.
From Rosenberg M, Lamba S, Misra S. Palliative medicine and geriatric emergency care: challenges, opportunities, and basic principles. Clin Geriatr Med 2013;29(1):1–29; with permission.

Box 1
Twelve primary palliative care skills for emergency providers

- Assessment of illness trajectory
- Determination of prognosis, communicate bad news
- Interpretation and formation of an advance care plan
- Family presence during resuscitation
- Symptom management (both pain and nonpain)
- Withdrawal and withholding of life-sustaining treatments
- Management of imminently dying patients
- Identify and implement hospice and palliative care referrals and care plans
- Understanding of ethical and legal issues pertinent to end-of-life care
- Display spiritual and cultural competency
- Management of the dying child

From Quest TE, Marco CA, Derse AR. Hospice and palliative medicine: new subspecialty, new opportunities. Ann Emerg Med 2009;54(1):95; with permission.

---

of history, physical examination, and medical decision making have been identified (**Box 2**). When patients present with a serious life-threatening illness, patients may be identified for primary palliative care intervention or subspecialty level consultation services based on clinical triggers (see **Table 1**). Several patients will present near the end of life in need of acute pain and nonpain symptom management. Hospice care may be appropriate directly from the ED.

CARE OF PATIENTS IN NEED OF OR UNDER A HOSPICE SYSTEM OF CARE

Patients who have already established hospice care often present to the ED. This population requires careful attention to the goals of care with a match of diagnostic and therapeutic interventions accordingly.

The first step in crafting a plan for these patients is recognizing why they presented to the ED. It is incorrect to assume that their presence in the ED indicates a desire for new investigative interventions and treatments but should be interpreted as an

---

Box 2
Key questions for primary palliative care assessment in the ED

- What are the acute medical issues and are they potentially reversible?
- What would most likely be the patients' status after treatment?
- What is the patients' recent performance level, the extent of the underlying disease, and the overall prognosis?
- What are the burdens of any treatments that could be offered?
- What are the patients'/surrogates' wishes when informed of the potential benefits and burdens of the treatment plan?

From Rosenberg M, Lamba S, Misra S. Palliative medicine and geriatric emergency care: challenges, opportunities, and basic principles. Clin Geriatr Med 2013;29(1):10; with permission.

opportunity to discuss any unmet needs. Reasons that these patients present to the ED include[11]

- Uncontrolled symptoms, such as pain, nausea, vomiting, or dyspnea
- Malfunction of a medical device (ie, gastrostomy tube dislodged)
- Emotional or existential distress on reflection of impending loss of life reflected as a change in the patients' acceptance of their condition
- Social stressors, such as a caregiver being unable or unwilling to provide care
- Poor communication with hospice staff and lack of understanding of services that hospice can provide in the nonacute hospital setting
- Desire to not die in the home setting: caregiver or cultural concerns of a home death
- Fear of the death process
- Lack of communication between caregivers of the goals of care

After identifying the factors that led patients receiving hospice care to come to the ED, a care plan may be crafted. The health care provider who sees hospice patients in the ED should

- Identify the patients' and families' goal and target interventions to meet that goal.
- Make recommendations on what would and would NOT help achieve these goals.
- Treat any distressing physical symptoms; if the goal is comfort, be as aggressive as necessary to address the distress.
- After intervening on any acute symptom that patients may have, it is important to coordinate early with the patients' hospice agency. It is important to be mindful of the fact that the hospice agency is financially responsible for all medical costs related to the terminal illness.
- Limit any diagnostic interventions, imaging, or laboratory tests that do not aid in accomplishing the patients' goals.
- Identify the surrogate decision maker, and do not assume that the person at the bedside with the patients is the legal decision maker.
- Identify explicitly where patients would like to ultimately die.
- Assess any cultural or spiritual issues that may have contributed to the patients presenting to the ED.
- Engage the inpatient palliative care consult team if available to assist with disposition and management.
- Coordinate disposition with the hospice agency. Hospice agencies can arrange for 24-hour professional support in the home setting if symptoms are difficult to control or if death is imminent.

For select patients, referral from the ED directly to hospice in an outpatient setting may be appropriate. Families of patients who died while in hospice have identified delays to hospice referral as a source of distress; of those who thought that they were referred to hospice too late, half thought that the barrier to earlier hospice services was physicians.[12] A sequence of steps can be undertaken to initiate hospice referrals from the emergency department. In most communities hospice referrals can be completed same or next day including weekends.[13]

- Assess Medicare hospice eligibility: Patients must have a prognosis of 6 months or less if the disease runs its usual course, and the patients' goals must be in alignment with the hospice philosophy.
- Discuss hospice as an option with the patients' physicians.
- Assess whether the goals of the patients are consistent with hospice.

- Introduce hospice to the patients, families, and all surrogates.
- Make a referral and write orders to a hospice agency.
- Ensure that the patients AND the surrogates understand the plan.
- If hospice enrollment is appropriate, but cannot be arranged in a timely manner, consider whether the patients can be safely cared for at home for 1 to 2 days without extra services. If so, write necessary prescriptions and discharge the patients. If not, admit the patients until a discharge plan can be crafted.

CLINICAL OUTCOMES

The trajectory of care initiated in the ED often determines the subsequent plans of action. The benefits of initiating palliative care from the ED may include alignment of patients' goals with the provider care plan, improved symptom control and quality of life, improved changes of access to earlier hospice and palliative care, decreased hospital and/or intensive-care-unit (ICU) length of stay, and improved overall health care utilization. The Integration of Palliative Care into Emergency Medicine: the Improving Palliative Care in Emergency Medicine collaboration is one online resource that is available to increase implementation palliative care for EM providers (http://www.capc.org/ipal/ipal-em).[14]

The evidence suggests that patients who are identified in the ED may have a high symptom burden and, when admitted from the ED to a palliative care unit, may have increased symptom control as well as increased likelihood of survival.[15] The average length of hospital stay of patients who receive a formal palliative care consult in the ED may be reduced.[16–18]

STRATEGIES TO IMPROVE PALLIATIVE CARE WITHIN THE EMERGENCY DEPARTMENT

Strategies to improve palliative care within the ED include

- Increase the number of palliative care consults initiated from the ED.
- Educate EM physicians on palliative care interventions that they themselves can use.
- Develop systems-based interventions within the ED, such as the creation of formal protocols under which palliative care consults are initiated.
- Integrate computer-generated triggers in an electronic medical record to flag possible patients for whom a palliative care approach would be warranted.

In order to increase the number of consults initiated from the ED, several approaches have been implemented. One approach is the formal identification of a champion within the department to spearhead palliative care initiatives. As palliative care is a multidisciplinary approach, there are many individuals who could serve as the champion, including an advanced-practice provider (nurse practitioner or physician assistant), a chaplain, nurse, or social worker. The impact of an ED palliative care champion can be substantial.[19] Rosenberg and Rosenberg[20] demonstrated that the effects of the champion model can greatly enhance an ED initiative with timely consultations by a variety of ED providers.

COMPLICATIONS AND CONCERNS

Barriers exist regarding the implementation of palliative care core principles and practice in the ED. Identified barriers include

- The perception that palliative care takes too much time
- Fear of litigation if interventions are withheld

- Lack of access to medical records or advanced care planning documents or an inability of patients to otherwise communicate what their goals are
- Availability of palliative care consults in the ED, although even in centers with robust palliative care consult teams, there is still marked underuse of this service in the ED[21]
- Lack of privacy/physical design layout of the ED not conducive to palliative care approach[22]
- Sense of conflict between mission of ED and palliative care[9]
- Failure to recognize which patients may benefit from a palliative care consult[23,24]
- A sense of discomfort with withholding or withdrawing life-sustaining interventions
- Inexperience with leading discussions regarding options that may include palliative or hospice care
- A significant percentage of residents never receive direct supervision or observation when conducting family meetings or delivering bad news and suffer from a sense of failure or guilt when caring for dying patients[25]
- Lack of knowledge of basic palliative care interventions[26]

EDUCATION IN PALLIATIVE CARE FOR EMERGENCY PROVIDERS

Palliative care has been identified as an area of opportunity for improvement in the curricula of emergency care providers. Emergency clinicians often lack basic palliative care skills, such as communicating options regarding hospice and managing basic opiate conversions. Fortunately, these shortcomings are found to be responsive to education. With only 4 hours of training regarding hospice, inpatient hospice referrals in one ED increased 88%; this increase was sustained 6 months after the formal training.[26] The Education in Palliative and End-of-life Care group-Emergency Medicine project has tailored series of courses for EM providers that aim to teach how to perform a rapid palliative assessment in the ED setting, how to formulate trajectories and prognoses, care of patients with cancer, communication strategies, family witnessed resuscitation, and techniques to teach these skills to other EM providers.[27]

SUMMARY

Palliative care in the ED is an expanding area of opportunity to deliver high-quality multidimensional care that is often more in alignment with the wishes of patients who are facing serious, potentially life-threatening diseases. There are a myriad of patient-centered benefits to integration of palliative care in the ED, including higher quality of life, better quality of death, improved symptom management, decreased rates of prolonged grief of family members, and a higher chance that patients' goals and physician care plans are in alignment. Further, there are significant benefits to the health care system with early delivery of palliative care, including reduced costs, reduced hospital length of stay, and reduced ICU admissions.

There remain a variety of barriers to the implementation of palliative care programs within the ED; however, there are strategies to overcome these barriers, such as formal education, identification of champions, and systems-based modifications.

REFERENCES

1. Wong J, Gott M, Frey R, et al. What is the incidence of patients with palliative care needs presenting to the emergency department? A critical review. Palliat Med 2014;28:1197–205.

2. Barbera L, Taylor C, Dudgeon D. Why do patients with cancer visit the emergency department near the end of life? CMAJ 2010;182(6):563–8.

3. Available at: http://www.cdc.gov/nchs/ahcd/web_tables.htm. Accessed October 31, 2014.

4. Delgado-Guay MO, Kim YJ, Shin SH, et al. Avoidable and unavoidable visits to the emergency department among patients with advanced cancer receiving outpatient palliative care. J Pain Symptom Manage 2014. [Epub ahead of print].

5. Grudzen CR, Stone SC, Morrison RS. The palliative care model for emergency department patients with advanced illness. J Palliat Med 2011;14(8):945–50.

6. SMith AK, McCarthy E, Weber E, et al. Half of older Americans seen in emergency department in last month of life; most admitted to hospital, and many die there. Health Aff (Millwood) 2012;31:1277–85.

7. Shearer FM, Rogers IR, Monterosso L, et al. Understanding emergency department staff needs and perceptions in the provision of palliative care. Emerg Med Australas 2014;26(3):249–55.

8. Bradley V, Burney C, Hughes G. Do patients die well in your emergency department? Emerg Med Australas 2013;25(4):334–9.

9. Stone SC, Mohanty S, Grudzen CR, et al. Emergency medicine physicians' perspectives of providing palliative care in an emergency department. J Palliat Med 2011;14(12):1333–8.

10. Available at: http://www.acep.org/Clinical—Practice-Management/ACEP-Announces-List-of-Tests-As-Part-of-Choosing-Wisely-Campaign/. Accessed October 31, 2014.

11. Lamba S, Quest TE, Weissman DE. Emergency department management of hospice patients #246. J Palliat Med 2011;14:1345–6.

12. Schockett ER, Teno JM, Miller SC, et al. Late referral to hospice and bereaved family member perception of quality of end-of-life care. J Pain Symptom Manage 2005;30:400–7.

13. Lamba S, Quest TE, Weissman DE. Initiating a hospice referral from the emergency department #247. J Palliat Med 2011;14:1346–7.

14. Lamba S, DeSandre PL, Todd KH, et al. Integration of palliative care into emergency medicine: the Improving Palliative Care in Emergency Medicine (IPAL-EM) Collaboration. J Emerg Med 2014;46(2):264–70.

15. Shin SH, Hui D, Chisholm GB, et al. Characteristics and outcomes of patients admitted to the acute palliative care unit from the emergency center. J Pain Symptom Manage 2014;47(6):1028–34.

16. Wu FM, Newman JM, Lasher A, et al. Effects of initiating palliative care consultation in the emergency department on inpatient length of stay. J Palliat Med 2013; 16(11):1362–7.

17. Hanson LC, Usher B, Spragens L, et al. Clinical and economic impact of palliative care consultation. J Pain Symptom Manage 2008;35:340–6.

18. May P, Normand C, Morrison RS. Economic impact of hospital inpatient palliative care consultation: review of current evidence and directions for future research. J Palliat Med 2014;17:1054–63.

19. Waugh DG. Palliative care project in the emergency department. J Palliat Med 2010;13(8):936.

20. Rosenberg M, Rosenberg L. Integrated model of palliative care in the emergency department. West J Emerg Med 2013;14(6):633–6.

21. Grudzen CR, Hwang U, Cohen JA, et al. Characteristics of emergency department patients who receive a palliative care consultation. J Palliat Med 2012; 15(4):396–9.

22. Glajchen M, Lawson R, Homel P, et al. A rapid two-stage screening protocol for palliative care in the emergency department: a quality improvement initiative. J Pain Symptom Manage 2011;42(5):657–62.
23. Zalenski R, Courage C, Edelen A, et al. Evaluation of screening criteria for palliative care consultation in the MICU: a multihospital analysis. BMJ Support Palliat Care 2014;4(3):254–62.
24. Ouchi K, Wu M, Medairos R, et al. Initiating palliative care consults for advanced dementia patients in the emergency department. J Palliat Med 2014;17:346–50.
25. Schroder C, Heyland D, Jiang X, et al. Educating medical residents in end-of-life care: insights from a multicenter survey. J Palliat Med 2009;12:459–70.
26. DeVader TE, Jeanmonod R. The effect of education in hospice and palliative care on emergency medicine residents' knowledge and referral patterns. J Palliat Med 2012;15(5):510–5.
27. Emmanuel LL, Quest TE, editors. The EPEC project. The Education in Palliative and End-of-life Care for Emergency Medicine (EPEC-EM) curriculum. Chicago: Northwestern University; 2008.

Index

Note: Page numbers of article titles are in **boldface** type.

A

Acetaminophen, 162, 202
Acupuncture, in pain management, 179, 180
Ageism, and communication, 232–233
Aging, demographic shift toward, 283
Aging population, and causes of morbidity and mortality, 254
Analgesia, use, misuse, and death, 199–200, 201

B

Bone pain, metastatic, prevention of, 163–164
    treatment of, 164
Bowel obstruction, 170
Brain death, 274
    determination of perceptions of health policies and, 275

C

Cancer, fatigue related to, 180
    intertwining of belief systems and, 286–287
    pain management in, 155
Cancer survival rates, in Middle East, 283–284
Care process, assessment of, cultural differentiation and, 284
Chronic disease, palliative care and, 284
    risk of, longevity and, 283
Commuication(s), barriers to, characteristics contributing to, 220
    family involvement in, 238–239
    information provision in, 221–222
    information tailoring in, 222
Communication(s), ageism and, 232–233
    as diagnostic and therapeutic tool, 234
    by professional in palliative care, **231–252**
    decision making and enabling of, 223–225
    discussions of, prognosis in, 227–238
    emphathic, 220–221
    excellent, importance of, 232
    family meeting for, facilitating of, 239–241
    focused conversation and, 233–236
    goals of patient and, 223, 224
    questions to open conversations, 235

Clin Geriatr Med 31 (2015) 305–310
http://dx.doi.org/10.1016/S0749-0690(15)00021-X
0749-0690/15/$ – see front matter © 2015 Elsevier Inc. All rights reserved.

Printed and bound by CPI Group (UK) Ltd, Croydon, CR0 4YY

03/10/2024

01040490-0014